The Difference We Make

Reflections on Lessons Learned Working in Community Mental Health

Celeste Charpentier Greene

Illustrated by James Irons

The Difference We Make: Reflections on
Lessons Learned Working in Community Mental Health

Visit our website at**www.StillwaterPress.com** for more information.

First Stillwater River Publications Edition.

ISBN: 978-1-968548-97-1

Library of Congress Control Number: 2026905547

1 2 3 4 5 6 7 8 9 10
Written by Celeste Charpenier Greene.
Illustrated by James Irons.
Cover photographs by JimmyC (front) and Water Shining (back) / Adobe Stock.
Published by Stillwater River Publications, West Warwick, RI, USA.

Publisher's Cataloging-in-Publication
(Provided by Cassidy Cataloguing Services, Inc.)
Names: Greene, Celeste Charpentier, author. |
Irons, James, illustrator.
Title: The difference we make : reflections on lessons learned working in community mental health / Celeste Charpentier Greene ; illustrated by James Irons.
Description: First Stillwater River Publications edition. |
West Warwick, RI, USA : Stillwater River Publications, [2026]
Identifiers: LCCN: 2026905547 | ISBN: 9781968548971 (paperback)
Subjects: LCSH: Greene, Celeste Charpentier. | Community mental health personnel. | Community mental health services. | Mentally ill. |
LCGFT: Autobiographies. | Anecdotes.
Classification: LCC: RC440.8 .G74 2026 | DDC: 362.22092--dc23

You cannot do all the good the world needs but
the world needs all the good you can do.

—Jana Stanfield,
songwriter and educator

Contents

Author's Disclaimer

"True enough." That is the phrase a client of mine used often during our counseling sessions. It is a good phrase, "true enough." I suppose that is what these reflections are: true enough. After retirement I found myself thinking of the many meaningful experiences that I had over the many years I spent working in community mental health. Then I started to write them down as memories became stories and made their way from my mind to paper. The stories revolved around the many lessons I learned over the years from clients and colleagues.

These stories are all true enough based on what my mind remembers. Though I have to admit that my brain is aging and sometimes misses things. However, the people are real and what happened did happen. The dialogue is fashioned to fit the narrative as I cannot recall verbatim what was actually said. However, the conversations are also true enough.

I have to admit that over the years when ridiculous things were happening, I wondered if I was being pranked. Was someone recording this to get a laugh at my expense? Would this be on YouTube or *America's Funniest Home Videos* or TikTok? Of course, no one was pranking me. There are no videos or tapes I can rely on to show exactly what happened, what was said and who was there. Though I can say for certain that when I was meeting with a client in my office or taking a ride with a client in the car, it was just the two of us.

What is real and true is the impact that the people I encountered through decades of working as a psychotherapist had on me. What is for certain is how grateful I am to have come to know them. I have tried to leave those who are in my stories as anonymous as I could, mostly by using a different name and attempting to be vague when possible. These stories are meant to reflect my appreciation and respect for clients and colleagues who are in these recollections. I apologize if anything written offends anyone I have included in these narratives. That was never the intention. The intention is to share a few stories about some rather fascinating people and experiences while staying "true enough" to the persons and experiences portrayed.

Introduction

A number of years ago, I was completely taken by a TV segment on CBS news by Steve Hartman called "Everybody Has a Story." Steve picked a random place in the US by throwing a dart at the map and then went to that place, found a phone book, and literally opened the book and put his finger on a name and called them. The first person to take up his offer to meet with him became the subject of that week's show. I found it fascinating and as each segment promised, everyone does have a story.

While I was never chosen by Steve Hartman and no darts or maps were involved in the writing of this book, I came to discover soon after I retired that I had a story to tell as well. Though, this is actually the story of how I was changed and became the person I am because of the stories other people shared with me. I had the blessing, privilege, and challenge to work in the field of community mental health for thirty-eight years. I was a mental health worker, sheltered workshop supervisor, program manager, residential counselor, substance use counselor, and psychotherapist to name a few different jobs over the years. In addition to these roles, there were so many other tasks that were taken on just so I could respond to the many needs of the persons entrusted to my care. Their stories entered into my own story as the people I worked with trusted me with their lives. What was shared with me changed me in ways that I could never have imagined. What follows is a collection of lessons about what I learned and experienced over those decades. You will be introduced to some of the wonderful people whom I had the privilege to work with over the years. In addition, each chapter will identify some of the lessons that I learned along the way.

I have always been a person of faith. Faith is not something that I can leave out of my life story. The stories presented reflect my belief that I was led and helped by the God who loves me and loves the clients and colleagues with whom I worked. Because what I believe in is so integral to how I experience life, I included my understanding of how God was a part of my work and the relationships that developed because of that work. It is how I have come to appreciate this most wonderful and humbling career that I had been blessed to have for as long as I did.

I hope that you enjoy these stories.

CHAPTER 1

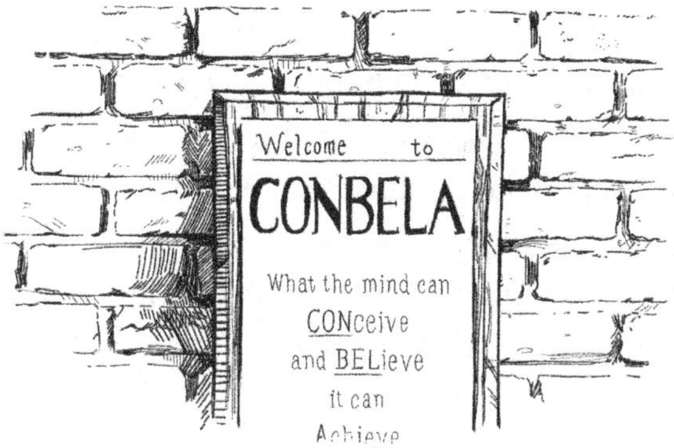
Welcome to
CONBELA
What the mind can
CONceive
and BELieve
it can

The Beginning

Life is a mystery. Things happen that we cannot anticipate, or even in the slightest way imagine. These things change the course, flavor, and color of our lives—forever. If you were to sit down with any human being in the world and ask them this one question "Is there any unexpected thing that happened to you that changed your life forever?" I guarantee that each person would have a surprising answer.

These unexpected things can be a positive event which might result in a lifelong, treasured relationship. Or it could be a devastating occurrence that turns life upside down and inside out. It can take one away from a hopeful path towards a life that involves struggle and challenge.

Most of us have experienced both kinds of events or relationships that have affected and influenced the course of our lives. This seems to be something most of us have in common. Life can be unpredictable.

As I reflect on what has influenced the direction of my life, a number of questions arise. How did my life become what it became? Is it chance, or coincidence, or fate? Is it the hand of God, or divine intervention? Since ancient times, humans have been working on an understanding of why things happen the way that they do. I do not attempt to suggest in any way that I have insights into the phenomenon. I only know that my life reflects the mystery and unpredictability that all of us experience. I also tend toward the belief that, somehow, God is a part of how my life story developed the way it did. This story begins with how life presented me a path that I would have never imagined or planned.

After college, I started my career path by working with adolescents. That is what I had planned and envisioned for myself before and through college. While there were many enjoyable moments and experiences working in the field of religious education with teens, in a few years it became apparent it wasn't quite the fit that I thought it would be.

There was a need for a different plan. Having no idea what that would be, I began to review and consider many options. I talked about it over and over with many friends and family members. Sometimes it entailed seeking out feedback from complete strangers. It was all part of the process of finding a new direction.

In the end, after much discussion and deliberation, I decided to apply to the Jesuit Volunteer Corps (JVC). It is a Catholic sponsored volunteer service organization for young adults. The core values of the organization are service to communities in need, putting faith into action, and finding opportunities to promote social justice while living in a community with other full-time volunteers. The earliest instance of the JVC was started in the 1950s by some dedicated Jesuit priests and nuns from the Sisters of St. Anne. These pioneering religious men and women decided to include a small group of recently graduated young men and women who had been students at the Catholic colleges where they were teaching. Their mission was to build and run a school for underserved communities in Alaska. It was a moving and successful experiment.

From these humble and unusual beginnings, the JVC was formed as the work was soon taken on by the Jesuit community of priests, who expanded the focus and service locations. Within a couple of decades, hundreds of JVC volunteers were working in communities all over the United States. The young adult volunteers worked in poorly resourced schools, ran soup kitchens, worked in homeless shelters, in mental health and medical care facilities, and so many other places. They worked as child care providers, educators, advocates for the homeless and abused, as well as many other types of service work. There were many opportunities to participate in work that can make a difference in the communities that were serviced all over the United States.

I applied to JVC Northwest. It included a year-long commitment to work full-time as a paid volunteer in a local service organization. JVC Northwest provided volunteers to work in the states of Oregon, Idaho, Montana, Washington, and Alaska. My application was accepted and I was going to be working in Seattle, Washington.

My first JVC destination was Portland, Oregon for orientation. After a week of meeting about a hundred other volunteers, learning about the mission and history of JVC, and generally enjoying ourselves, it was time to head out to our assignments. I had my car with me so, a couple of other volunteers who were also assigned to work in Seattle joined me for the drive up north.

After a three-hour drive north on Route I-5, we arrived in Seattle, Washington. Entering into the beauty of the northwest was incredible. We were surrounded by tall conifers, majestic snow-capped mountains, dazzling lakes, and Puget Sound, which actually looked like an ocean. It was all so gorgeous; I tried without success to get my head to spin completely around so I could take it all in all at once. Every day in Seattle I was amazed at how beautiful this part of the country is.

JVC provided the housing. The house where we lived was located just a couple blocks away from Garfield High School where Jimi Hendrix went. Our neighborhood was one of the more diverse areas within Seattle. We lived in a home typical of other homes in our area: a two-story clapboard yellow-and-brown structure with a small backyard and lots of steps to get to the front door in this very hilly neighborhood. Seattle is very hilly. Our neighbors were used to people moving in and out of the house as a new crew of young adults would arrive every August.

Living with other volunteers was an important part of the overall experience. I had six roommates. These incredible six young adults would be my surrogate family for twelve months. My housemates hailed from New York, Minnesota, Massachusetts, North Carolina, and one of my roommates had been born and raised in Haiti. Being the fourth of seven siblings, living with that many people was not much of a stretch for me. However, having the largest bedroom all to myself was an amazing bonus.

Except for me, all of my roommates had just graduated college, while I had been out of college for the past five years. That difference was quite significant as I found myself being the big sister in the room more often than I wished to be. I had already had a number of years living completely on my own with classes, teachers, and dorm rooms well in my past. They were just beginning to learn the lessons of independent adult living, more or less. Making adjustments and allowances for our individual needs and experiences was exactly the lesson I needed to learn from this living adventure. We all had some growing up to do, especially me. I am forever grateful for the challenges and support this communal living situation provided. Learning to laugh at my foibles and let go of things I needed to let go of—like being judgmental about how others choose to use their free time and whose turn it is to clean the kitchen—was exactly what I needed.

Despite our unique backgrounds and personalities, our little family was able to gel together. We all loved to laugh and bake and eat cookies. We found a way to work out decision-making and resolve differences, and our little house became a comfortable home away from home. We grew to be quite fond of each other. Many times, this group would be the supportive presence that made a positive difference as we all adjusted to our service work in a new and unfamiliar place. Of course, the cookies and the laughter were a big help.

JVC assigned each of us a job. My job would be working as a mental health worker in an adult day treatment/Clubhouse program for adults with chronic and persistent mental illness. With absolutely no previous experience, exposure, or understanding of mental illness, my first few weeks of work were overwhelming. I was the human version of a deer in headlights those first few weeks. I probably just stood there with a perplexed "What the heck?" or "Get me out of here!" kind of look on my face. Grown people were walking around in a kind of zombie state. Their movements were stiff and awkward. Many of them talked to themselves as they paced up and down hallways. They would not want to look at me and they would become uncomfortable if I looked at them. A few of the members, as the participants were called, would just stand there as if they were holding up the wall and if they moved, the wall would fall. Some members were very friendly. They would think nothing of coming into my personal space. They talked rapidly and it was not always clear what they were talking about.

Did the organizers at JVC realize they had chosen me for a job that I was not at all trained for or ready for? I felt overwhelmed, anxious and distressed. As I took the bus through Seattle back and forth from work those early days, I would head there in a cold sweat and return home staring blankly as I tried to figure out what planet I was on.

I was very much out of my element those first few weeks at CONBELA. That was the name of the agency where I worked. There was a large sign when you first entered the facility that read: **Welcome**

to CONBELA: What the mind can *CON*ceive and *BEL*ieve, it can *A*chieve. That was the motto and philosophy of the program. In time, an appreciation for that motto would come.

If I had not had the benefit of working with the most wonderful supervisors and coworkers, I am not sure I would have stayed. They patiently mentored me, providing much understanding, support, and guidance. They were tactfully encouraging so that the lessons needed to be learned could start to take hold. My coworkers and the psychiatrist we worked with provided training, valuable skill building and endless teaching through example. There was much to be learned about the different types of mental illness, about how medication can help and about how challenging this new phase of mental health treatment was. Every day I worked there I was stretched out of my comfort zone as I learned to be more patient, open, and accepting.

The most valuable lessons came from the members themselves. As part of my job, I was assigned to work with one of the clients/members. The person I was to work with was Tony. He was about six feet tall, with thick wavy brown hair and blue eyes which he rarely let anyone see.

Lanky and often disheveled, he was a loner and tended toward isolation as much as he could. I was told that he had paranoid schizophrenia and started to experience hallucinations and delusions in his early twenties. Tony was around twenty-eight years old when we met. I knew absolutely nothing about what he was experiencing and my initial attempts to connect with him and get to know him went absolutely nowhere. Standing in the hallway with his back to the wall was his usual activity. He would stand there for hours, mostly looking down at his feet, talking to himself.

When Tony wasn't hanging out by his favorite wall, he and I would be working in the kitchen making salad. As we broke apart the lettuce and cut carrots, celery, and tomatoes, I would try to talk with him about whatever I could come up with at the time. There was not much response from him and he appeared to be quite uncomfortable as I tried to involve him in conversation. As soon as the salad was ready, he was out of the kitchen and trying to be as far away from me as he could. Our initial attempts at connecting were painful for me and for him. I felt like such a dunce. There was nothing I could pull from my past relationships or experiences that were helpful at CONBELA. My supervisors and coworkers encouraged me to be patient and just keep trying.

One day, as Tony was standing with his back to the wall, I decided that I would just do what he was doing. So, I stood with my back to the wall and looked down at my feet. We stood there together for quite a while not saying anything to each other. After a time as I continued to look down at my feet I said to him, "Tell me something about your family." With his eyes also looking down at his feet, he started to tell me about his family and his upbringing.

Whoa! What is happening here? I thought to myself as he shared about his brothers and he growing up in a Seattle suburb. I was blown away as he volunteered personal information about himself. My eyes welled up with tears as he shared about himself. We did it. We started to make a connection with each other. It took a good two to three months for something to happen, but happen it did. Something about making that first connection hooked me. From that time on, I became completely fascinated with mental health work.

I wanted to learn more and my curiosity about mental illness and mental health treatment led me to ask questions, to reach out, to find ways to connect. I learned how to listen and help members to tell me what they could of their life stories. Working at CONBELA led me to the most wonderful human beings I have ever met. I came to love the work and love the members. There seemed to be something honest and genuine about members as I came to know them. There was never any pretense or game playing. However, there was the challenge of disability, the loss of what could have been, and the reality of struggle, isolation, and poverty. As relationships grew and developed, I found myself tapping into compassion and a desire to understand and accept people just for who they are. Before I knew it, I began to feel at home working in community mental health.

It was the mid-1980s. This was a time when treatment for adults with chronic mental illness was going through drastic changes. State institutions for the mentally ill were being emptied and laws were being enacted to provide less restrictive housing back in local communities where their families lived. Vocational opportunities and social integration were happening in states all over the US. Treatment and rehabilitation opportunities became available in the form of community mental health centers and private rehabilitation agencies. Medical treatment for chronic mental illness improved as new pharmaceuticals were developed. Medications continued to have a lesser sedating effect on members than in years past. As a society, there was a commitment to undo the practices of state institutions that "warehoused" the mentally ill.

People who had been confined there for years now had a pathway to reenter into society.

Programs like CONBELA were providing an opportunity to help reintegrate the mentally ill back into a society that had become unfamiliar to them after years of institutionalization. I learned to believe in the importance of making change happen in the most ordinary ways. We would cook a meal together, play Ping-Pong, or go for a walk. I helped members organize social events to celebrate a holiday or to commemorate the birthdays for the month. The agency ran a recycling business. We recycled paper, cardboard, glass, and metals. Members would take turns working in the business and learning some helpful work skills. Another part of my job was to work side by side with members helping to reacquaint them with a work environment. People who had been disempowered, put away and silenced, now were being given chances to claim back their lives, their voices, and their dignity. That was the work of "Conceiving," "Believing," and "Achieving." Most of the changes were small and unnoticeable in some ways, but quite remarkable in other ways. I felt very fortunate to be a part of this new movement. It was time to provide expanded opportunities for a group of people who had been quite forgotten. It was time for change.

That volunteer year changed my life forever. I found my own CONBELA experience. I began to think about and CONceive myself working in the field of mental health. I came to BELieve in the work and in the possibility of helpful change. From that came the start of plans to move in a new direction. I focused on ways to Achieve this newfound vision. I found my path, pursuing a career working with the mentally ill in community mental health that would last for decades.

For thirty-eight years my life was focused on working in a number of mental health facilities, including day treatment programs, Clubhouses, residences, a psychiatric hospital, adult correctional facilities, and a number of community mental health centers doing community outreach and office counseling. That one year of volunteer service work became a new beginning for me. I found a new way of conceiving a vision for myself, believing that this was the right path for me and working on making this vision not only a possibility but a reality.

The tongue-in-cheek motto for the Jesuit Volunteer Corps is "ruined for life." That is what happened to me. Before participating in the Jesuit Volunteer Corps, I was considering going back to school to study accounting or food science or something that would be considered a good job and pay well. My thinking before JVC was to have a good paying job and use time outside of work to volunteer and pursue interests that would support my beliefs and faith. While that life would have been just fine, I can't help but be grateful for joining JVC. Because of the experiences I had in that volunteer year, I was thinking very differently about where my life was heading. Whatever conventional and predictable vision I had for myself before JVC was far behind me in the rearview mirror of life. I felt a need and indeed a bit of a compulsion to devote my life to service, and in particular to being of service to those with mental illness. My former dreams were in ruins, but not in a bad way. In place of those dreams was an excitement about devoting myself to a population that I had absolutely no knowledge of pre-JVC. This new dream would become the focus and passion of my life moving forward.

CHAPTER 2

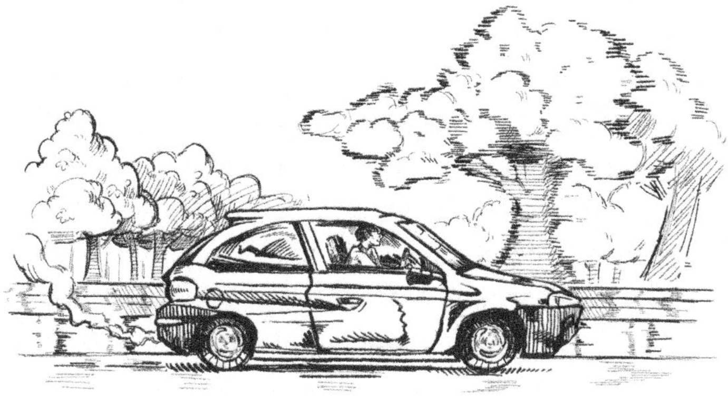

Leaving Things in Chaos

I spent much time thinking about and imagining what it would be like to work in the mental health treatment field. It meant going back to school to pursue a graduate degree in counseling psychology. After some research and checking out my options, Boston was chosen as the place to move for that education. While I still had to actually choose a school and program, it was clear that Boston made the most sense since there were a number of reputable universities and colleges to choose from for graduate school. I was originally from the little state of Rhode Island, so, in a way I was going back home.

I was living in Seattle, Washington at the time, so I packed my little Chevy Geo with all that I had, got on Route 90, and headed east. Boston is the easternmost point on Route 90—a straight shot from west to east but also a three thousand-mile journey. It was a beautiful ride over mountains and plains and through villages and historic sites. The drive was absolutely beautiful.

However, there was going to be a little layover in Chicago. My oldest sister was getting married that summer, so I had to get a move on. I had to get to Chicago in time to be there for her wedding in August of 1986. As it so happened, all of my six siblings and I were going through major transitions as we met in Chicago that summer.

My oldest sister, Elaine, was getting married. My next oldest sister, Cloe, would be leaving shortly for Bolivia in South America to pursue missionary work. Maggie, my third oldest sister, was moving from Denver to Vermont. I was moving from Seattle to Boston. My younger sister, Simone, was moving from New York to Boston. My younger brother Ron, and his wife Jan, also arrived in Chicago with their truck loaded with their belongings as they moved from Massachusetts to Oregon. And my youngest brother, JP, had just graduated high school and was about to start college. Even my parents were experiencing one of the biggest changes in their adult lives as they were about to be without children in the home for the first time in thirty-four years.

Those few days in Chicago were memorable. We all went to a Cubs game, explored a little bit of Chicago, and participated in a lovely wedding ceremony at Loyola University, where my brother-in-law, Jim, was teaching. All seven of us were on the verge of new adventures and opportunities. That wedding was an incredible experience as all of us celebrated how love not only brought us all together but would continue to hold us together no matter where life was taking us.

I arrived in Boston at the very beginning of September with much hope and anxiety. The first thing was to find a roommate and an affordable apartment. That worked out very well and within a week, I had a wonderful roommate and a beautiful apartment in the city. Shortly after I settled into my new apartment, it was time to look for work in the mental health field. Working and saving a bit of money was crucial if graduate school was going to happen. My first year in Boston afforded me that chance.

Looking through want ads in newspapers was the way to find

work at the time. So, one Sunday morning while combing through *The Boston Globe*, I came upon a want ad for a program offering a holistic approach to mental health rehabilitation and treatment. The ad indicated that this program combined vocational opportunities with holistic approaches to mental health treatment, such as attention to physical, social, and spiritual needs. Intriguing! Intuitively I knew, thanks to my limited experience, that when someone is diagnosed with a major mental illness, the whole person is affected. I wanted to know more about this place. What kind of holistic approach to mental health treatment was being offered? I sent in my résumé immediately. Astonishingly, I received a callback within days and an interview was scheduled.

I was living in the Jamaica Plain section of Boston, which is in the southwest corner of the city. My interview was in Lynn, Massachusetts, northeast of Boston and about twenty miles away from Jamaica Plain. I traversed the city, headed northeast on Route 1 over the Tobin Bridge and eventually into the city of Lynn on the North Shore. It was a lovely drive into the city—the area had a vibrant mill community at one time, known especially for shoe manufacturing. I found my way to the agency, Community Health and Alternative Opportunity Services. A white clapboard building with wide front steps and a redbrick foundation, I think it had been a union hall back in the day.

Of course, I had on my best interview outfit—a sleek skirt and nice blouse with a stylish jacket. I hoped that I looked just professional enough for this interview. However, I approached the building feeling a bit anxious and unsure. It is hard to put yourself out there to people that are unfamiliar. Would I be able to sell myself to them? I had no background in holistic treatment of any kind. Nor did I have any formal schooling in psychology. Would what I had to offer be what they were looking for in a work candidate?

Entering the building I was greeted by Kathy, one of the founders of the agency, and her German shepherd. Appearing to be in her late thirties, she was attractive and also dressed professionally in a skirt and blouse. Her dog stood close by, protective and alert. He scared me a bit so I held out my hand for him to sniff and give the okay for me to enter. Kathy had an easy and approachable way about her as she began to conduct the job interview and helped me to feel somewhat at ease. She was obviously proud of what she and her cofounder Jeff had put together as she began to describe how the agency came about. She had studied psychology and worked in psychiatric hospitals and mental health agencies for a bit. Her cofounder Jeff had a degree in rehabilitation and was well trained in helping those with disabilities to use work to restore abilities and opportunities. They had met when they both worked at the same agency a number of years ago. They discovered that they had similar interests and approaches. Both she and Jeff had become interested in holistic approaches including using the arts, nutrition, body work, and attention to the inner person. They combined their interests and efforts and started their own agency.

We met in her office and she began by explaining how the program worked. The program they created incorporated rehabilitation elements in the form of a sheltered workshop and mental health treatment groups that combined her interest in holistic health and her belief that the clients needed an approach that addressed all of their needs—mind, body, and spirit. She was most enthusiastic about this approach.

I tried my best to focus on her presentation, asking questions and answering her questions, as her German shepherd approached me while I sat across from her desk. He started to sniff around, getting closer and closer until he could not keep his nose out of my crotch!! He was way too persistent obeying whatever urge was going on in his brain and nose—he would not be distracted. Kathy did not seem to notice at all as I petted the dog and tried to hold his head away from my personal areas. It was most unsettling. Not only that, he was shedding and slobbering all over my interview skirt. I had other interviews to attend that week! What to do? Do I say something? Should I ask if her dog would like to be closer to her? Should I ask for a doggie treat or should I just jump up and create a scene? I did none of those things as I took my cue from Kathy and pretended that nothing was out of the ordinary.

I do not know how I maintained my composure during that fifteen-minute interview in her office. Needless to say, I was more than ready to get up and take a tour of the building when Kathy offered. Luckily, Fido was put into his crate while we had our tour. Kathy explained that she kept him away from the clients because he could be quite distracting to them. No kidding!!

We had an interesting tour of the facility. She took her time walking me through the building and showing off what she was proud of. I have to admit that the program she and Jeff had created was brilliant. In the basement, at ground level, was the sheltered workshop where twenty to thirty adults could work and get paid for piece work. It was a large room with worktables set up on either side of the room. Two to three workers could sit at a station at a time. At one end of the room was another worktable centered in the middle of the room where the work supervisor had their station. The room was well lit, which was very important as there were no windows in this part of the building. There was a positive feel to the space. Even though I was there outside of work hours, it felt comfortable.

Behind the work floor was a full-size kitchen and dining area. A meal program was provided for clients and staff. The agency offered a macrobiotic lunch three times a week. The chef also offered opportunities to teach clients healthy food options and food preparation as part of their recovery program.

Mental health treatment took place on the main floor in ample and well-lit treatment rooms that focused on group therapy and expressive arts groups. Large windows in both treatment rooms created an airy, pleasant vibe. The decor featured positive sayings, original artwork, and colorful seating. There was also a space for movement and massage services that helped clients have a better recovery from the effects of mental health medications on their body.

As we made our way back to her office Kathy shared that she was quite excited about my interest in the agency. In fact, she offered me the job! I actually said yes on the spot. My job would be to coordinate the sheltered workshop and after I learned more about how treatment groups worked, I would also participate in that work.

"Welcome to CHAOS," Kathy said happily. She noticed the perplexed look on my face. She said slowly, "**C**ommunity **H**ealth and **A**lternative **O**pportunity **S**ervices: CHAOS." I remembered the sign on the building with the same words.

"Oh, how clever," I responded with a catch in my throat. How could I have missed that??? The acronym for their program was CHAOS! I had just agreed to be a staff person at CHAOS! What was I getting myself into??!! Doesn't "chaos" stand for things being all muddled and ridiculous?

I took myself and my slobbered-over interview skirt back to Jamaica Plain. I was partly relieved that I had a job and partly freaked out that I had no clue about holistic approaches to treatment. I had no idea what a macrobiotic diet was or what expressive arts therapy was. In addition, I had no idea how to run a sheltered workshop. Besides that, why would anyone name a mental health program CHAOS? Maybe that was not as humorous as they imagined. I would soon find out.

Our team was made up of wonderful people who lived life in their own lane. They were innovative individuals who shared their endless creativity with clients and staff alike. They were open and accepting and so supportive. Influenced by the New Age movement, conversations in the staff room centered around topics like harmonic convergences, spiritual consciousness, differences between vegan and vegetarian, how to use crystals and flower essences, and going for retreats at Kripalu in the Berkshires, a center for yoga and holistic health. I was not well-versed in any of those topics. Hence, it wasn't easy for me to participate in many conversations in the staff room, but I did find them quite fascinating.

The expressive arts therapist became my supervisor. She was amazing at both. She had an undergraduate degree in art and a master's degree in expressive therapies through Lesley College (now Lesley University) in Cambridge, Massachusetts. Expressive therapists are licensed mental health counselors with specialized training using expressive arts such as drawing, painting, poetry, acting, etc., in their work. They integrate treatment strategies using creativity, imagination, expression, and experience to treat the whole person—mind, body, and spirit. My supervisor ran all sorts of expressive art groups using drawing, painting, clay, writing, and verbal expression. She also did some individual work as well using a number of different art mediums. She helped clients to connect with and bring out into the open things for which they could not find words. I learned so much from her about the many ways to listen to clients. Most importantly, I learned to be observant about the whole person.

There were two other expressive arts therapists who also worked on staff while I was there. They added their own flare to their work. They were both performance artists who taught us how to express ourselves using our words, our emotions, and our bodies. They were not at all shy about being noticed. One was a slam poet who loved to perform before an audience using much emotion and drama. She was incredible at helping clients and staff connect with their own poetic selves. The other staff member was an actor. She taught the value of finding the many versions of ourselves through voice and response. It was amazing.

Our movement/licensed massage therapist was a hoot. She was a hugger by nature and did amazing work with clients to help address the side effects of the psychiatric medications they were taking. Medication would leave many of them feeling stiff and uncomfortable. Some clients had involuntary movements in their legs or face that were noticeable and discomforting. Those movement groups were very well received. She also provided individual massages to clients to address their particular physical body needs. Outside of work, she was dedicated to meditation and spent many weekends at Kripalu in the Berkshires or attending a harmonic convergence gathering. She always had a hilarious story about her adventures.

Our chef was a skinny Italian guy from Boston who was just incredibly talented. He could make a killer lasagna without using dairy, meat, or gluten products!!!! WHAT???? He was passionate about making vegetarian food that tasted and looked good. He was especially committed to creating familiar meals that were as good as what we were used to. He was determined to make his traditional Italian dishes as authentic to the eye and taste as possible while using tofu, gluten free, and nondairy products. Most of the time, he succeeded. What was especially endearing was his Boston accent as he would describe the meal of the day:

"Okay yooz guys, Paak (park) your bottoms in your cheers (chairs) and get ready for a lunch that will knock your socks off!"

You get the gist.

I also worked a lot with Jeff, the cofounder of CHAOS. What a great guy and mentor! He was smart, funny, and had very good business sense. His job was to make connections with businesses to subcontract work that our clients could do in the workshop. He was very supportive of me as I had a lot to learn. I did have a little bit of exposure to rehabilitation work back in Seattle but I had no experience coordinating and executing a rehabilitation program. He taught me how to work with our clients and how to adjust the work so that they could succeed and make some decent money. I really appreciated this training. It meant a lot to me that our clients did well in their work, felt good about what they were doing, and were pleased that they were making some money. We had contracts with a local business and prepared eyeglass cases for the factory to finish them off for sale. We also did some bulk mail work, filling and stamping envelopes for two nonprofit agencies.

What was much appreciated was Jeff's awareness of my pragmatic approach to the work. Because of his background in business and his education in rehabilitation, he was the more practical one of the duo with Cathy. He and I were also a good fit because we were the more grounded people on the team as a whole. Jeff helped me to make the connections between the practical needs of work and the abstract needs of each client. It helped me to recognize the importance of the whole person in treatment and healing. In addition, Jeff and I had a compatible sense of humor. He was especially good at helping me not to take myself too seriously. Needed laughter at just the right time was always appreciated.

I really enjoyed working with the clients. I got to spend more time with them than other staff so we got to know each other very well. They taught me about just being real and "in the moment." I probably had more in common with the clients than with my coworkers. We tended to be less affected by New Age influences. The clients definitely appreciated that I could talk about the best places to go for a hamburger or what was happening with the Red Sox or Boston Bruins.

I also was able to help them incorporate what they were learning in their groups into the work they did in the workshop. How interesting is that! For instance, the movement therapist helped with how to sit to avoid pain and improve stamina. On the work floor, we would integrate things learned from groups. Following a therapy group session, clients would return to the work floor with new skills they wanted to integrate into their work. This showed up in improved concentration and focus. What a benefit that with mutual support, clients could put what they learned immediately into practice.

I also learned a lot more about mental illness. Clients had numerous distractions and challenges doing the work because of their mental health symptoms. Persons with thought disorders, like schizophrenia or other psychotic disorders, had a difficult time maintaining concentration. They would talk to themselves, or start to laugh over something only they could hear. I discovered with their help that reaching out once in a while to gently and respectfully bring them back to present reality seemed to be helpful. Clients with mood disorders like depression or bipolar disorder often just needed space to find their way as best as they could from their inner ups and downs. For them the work was very helpful in adjusting their moods, offering something to focus on that helped a bit in managing challenging thoughts and feelings. With them a little side conversation and encouragement became very useful in helping them to do well in completing work assignments.

The client who presented the biggest challenge to me on the work floor was a man with obsessive-compulsive disorder. Because of his OCD, he had multiple challenges with the demands of the work. It was almost impossible for him to move from one completed piece of work to the next. When working on the eyeglass cases he would apply his adhesive piece, then take it off and reapply the same piece over and over again. He wanted so desperately to succeed in the work but was struggling mightily. He loved attending the groups and we tried to apply what he was learning in groups to his time on the work floor. Some days he did okay but most days he would complete twenty or thirty pieces to everyone else completing hundreds of pieces in a day. He rarely missed a day of work. We worked together tirelessly to figure out ways to help him address his OCD behaviors and improve his work performance. Applying the holistic approaches gleaned from groups became a daily experiment on the work floor. We used singing, meditation, and simple movement exercises, among a number of other approaches. Some were more successful than others. Fortunately, there were a number of days that his work performance improved noticeably. He taught me much about perseverance. He never gave up. He found ways to laugh at himself and his pleasant personality and sense of humor were appreciated by all of the other workers. We all loved him so dearly. Other workers encouraged him, assisted him, and treated him as a valuable member of our work community.

There were so many wonderful and unusual opportunities to learn about therapy and working in the field of mental health at CHAOS. I learned about holistic approaches to the many mental health challenges that affected clients, including using the arts, imagination, music, repetitive movement, meditation, breathing, positive encouragement, and active listening. For me, holistic approaches had many configurations that went well beyond New Age philosophies. If anything, the uniqueness of each of my colleagues helped me appreciate my own uniqueness. Staff were successful because they were true to themselves. They made time for their own self-healing and they made time to support their continued growth. Working at this agency helped me to be true to my own self as well. My upbringing, my faith, my interests, and my talents were what I needed to connect with in order to be a more effective clinician. I also learned from this experience to be sure that I always made time for my own continuing growth, self-care, and healing.

Within my first year of working at CHAOS, I decided on where I wanted to attend graduate school and made my application to Lesley College. I started graduate school while I was still working at CHAOS. I was accepted at Lesley College in Cambridge in the counseling psychology program in the holistic track. Clearly my work at CHAOS had a lot to do with that choice.

CHAOS is where I got my first paying job working in community mental health. I got myself into an experience that I could never have imagined. It was instrumental in preparing me both for graduate school studies and for my career working in mental health. Kathy took a chance hiring me because it was clear from the beginning that I was a bit different from other staff there.

Because of that, I did bring something that was valuable to their work. I felt appreciated because of my practicality and work ethic. It was what the sheltered workshop needed. I was a good fit for helping clients to improve work skills and set work goals for themselves. I was able to work closely with them to make the sheltered workshop a valuable experience for them. I learned to appreciate being true to myself and my own unique contributions; I needed to acknowledge my own value. I also learned that the holistic approach to mental health care is crucial to working in this field. Focusing on the whole person—mind, body, and spirit—brought a focus to my work that stayed with me throughout my career.

After two meaningful and formative years of working at CHAOS, it was time for me to say goodbye. I had completed my first year of graduate school and was getting ready to increase my class load and start an internship to complete the requirements for the master's program. There was no way that I could work full-time at CHAOS and manage graduate school and an internship at the same time. My notice was delivered and I would be leaving CHAOS at the end of August.

The graduate program at Lesley encouraged us to connect with our personal gifts and interests as a way to develop our counseling skills. Music has always been an important influence in my life. While playing musical instruments had been a part of my life for many years, writing and creating music were not. Yet, as I prepared to leave CHAOS, I found myself writing a goodbye song. The one and only time I sang the song out loud for others was during my last week there, right on the workshop floor. I sang to staff and clients with a shaky voice, clutching my guitar and hoping that I could get through it without making too much of a mess of it. I am not a performer so it had to come from my heart as I nervously got the words out and my fingers moved from chord to chord.

I called the song "Leaving Things In CHAOS." The song was my way of acknowledging what a blessing it was to work there. So many important early lessons about mental illness and treatment had been learned, including an appreciation of how a loving and sincere connection with clients and staff are an important part of all lessons. Another reality is that sometimes acknowledging change is needed does not mean that everything else needs to change. While CHAOS changed me, the program and experience of CHAOS did not have to change. Hence, another valuable lesson was to focus on the places where change is necessary and let go of the rest.

Here are the lyrics:

How did I end up here?
When I could have ended up there?
Who would have ever thought
That life could be so strange
And I would end up in CHAOS.
    So I'm leaving things in CHAOS.
    Leaving things just as they are.
    Acceptance brings a peaceful joy,
    Change is what brings growth
    And love is the gift that binds us all.
I hope for all of you the life you so deserve.
I wish for you the jobs you want and people who will care.
And when life presents its scary side and you feel all alone,
I pray you'll find the guiding hand of love deep in your soul.
    So I'm leaving things in CHAOS.
    Leaving things just as they are.
    Acceptance brings a peaceful joy,
    Change is what brings growth
    And love is the gift that binds us all.
So here's to you, my friends, for making my life real.
I'm glad I ended up here for the chance to love and feel,
The truth that I take with me on the road I travel on,
That God created life out of CHAOS.

So I'm leaving things in CHAOS
Leaving things just as they are.
Acceptance brings a peaceful joy,
Change is what brings growth
And love is the gift that binds us all.

And even though I never worked in the city of Lynn again nor had contact with CHAOS, clearly there is much that I took with me, much that stayed with me and much that influenced how my life progressed. This experience helped me to focus on how I learned, how I worked on my own healing, and how I was able to stay working in the field of mental health for decades to come, NO MATTER HOW CHAOTIC!

CHAPTER 3

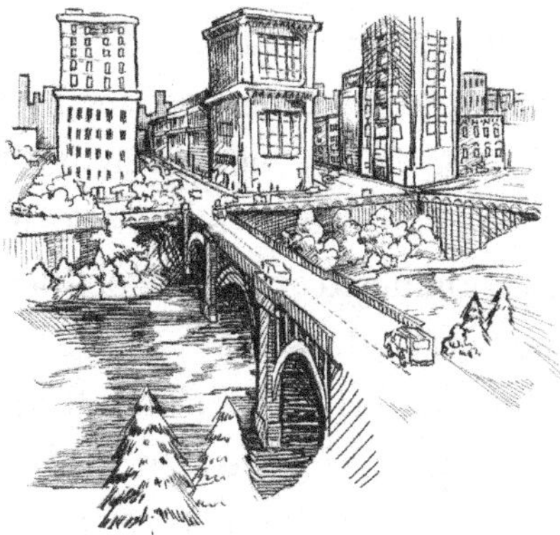

The Worst Week

How lucky I was to be hired so quickly after I completed my master's program. Finding a job was the challenge after graduation. Believe it or not, there are not that many graduate level positions in the field of community mental health. Most of the positions are for bachelor, associate degree, or high school education level of training. Positions that are most available involve direct service in group homes, job training, or day treatment programs. These include services like transporting clients, doing residential care, or assisting persons with social and vocational training. I was fortunate to have worked in some of these positions before finishing my master's program and came to appreciate the importance of everyone's contribution in providing community mental health services.

After grad school I was hired as a program manager for a Clubhouse program in Massachusetts. The Massachusetts Office of Mental Health Services had a very active and effective commitment to the Clubhouse philosophy and practice for rehabilitation services. The Clubhouse model was started in New York City by persons with chronic mental illness who wanted to have more influence and independence in their treatment and progress. In the beginning, Clubhouses were completely organized and run by peers—people with chronic and persistent mental illness. The members made the Clubhouse management decisions collectively. It proved to be a very interesting and successful approach to mental health treatment. The concept became institutionalized and some people without chronic mental illness became part of the staff.

Frankly, it helped to keep the program vibrant because there were more consistent resources to help fund and run worthwhile approaches to treatment. With the help of the State, there were active Clubhouses in almost every significant population area in Massachusetts.

I started to work in a Clubhouse in a busy city in Massachusetts with a long industrial history. As with so many of the industrialized cities in New England, there was a powerful river that flowed right through the city. The river was the source of its industrial focus and a symbol of the beauty of this part of New England.

I supervised about a dozen paid Clubhouse staff in our busy little agency. We were committed to the practice of all members who participated in services being involved in the day-to-day decisions about the Clubhouse. There were at least forty to sixty active members who participated at least three to four days a week and another fifty or so members that came at least weekly. Our philosophy incorporated practical work skills with a focus on the Clubhouse's community support for all of our members. We also offered members a chance to learn weaving. We had a weaving shop overseen by two staff persons with an art background. They taught members how to make gorgeous runners, place mats, shawls, and scarfs on wooden looms that were operated manually.

Overall, we hoped that we were helping to train our members for competitive employment. We had a very active job training focus. From Monday to Friday, members and staff were present to work on specific work needs right at the Clubhouse. We had a business crew, a maintenance crew, a food service crew, a snack bar crew, and the weaving studio. With a commitment to encouraging and supporting competitive employment, we also had a vocational specialist who worked with nearby businesses to find paid competitive work that our members could do. We also provided a drop-in space for social activities weekday evenings and on Saturdays and Sundays.

What always excited me most in any job I had was work that was anything but routine. I thrived on new experiences and daily challenges. The Clubhouse did not disappoint. In addition, I believe in the power of daily member involvement in decision-making. Giving anyone agency over their own life in as many ways as possible is a value I strongly support. For instance, if we needed to hire staff to work at the Clubhouse, members participated in the process of interviewing and hiring staff. Members also participated in decisions about how to run the different crews, such as deciding on menus for the week, being in charge of the newsletter, and going out with staff to the hardware store or the grocery store to purchase what was needed for the Clubhouse.

I worked hard and kept very busy with the management of the Clubhouse. There were so many enjoyable moments while there, as well as interesting people and growth-filled opportunities. Along with the weaving crew, I participated in local craft fairs where our weavers could showcase and sell their work to the public. How gratifying for them to receive so many compliments about the quality and beauty of their creations. I was very involved in helping to connect members with competitive work opportunities. Many hours were spent out in the community working side by side with a member who was learning a new job and needed some support and encouragement to succeed in their new position.

After working three years at the Clubhouse, I decided it was time for me to move on. I was missing the individual counseling work that I had been trained for in graduate school. The Clubhouse model was not set up to provide that type of experience for our members. Members had therapists, but not through the Clubhouse. They went to the community mental health center for that service. While members did come to me seeking that kind of support, it was not what I was there for, so I would help to make referrals for them to meet with their own individual therapists at the local community mental health center. In graduate school there were opportunities to provide individual counseling during my internship at a psychiatric hospital, which was challenging and fascinating. My heart began to yearn for the individual connections that psychotherapy provides. It was time for me to move into that type of work environment. As my last week of work approached, everyone, including me, was trying to deny the inevitable. I enjoyed the work there so much. The members and staff were the best people to work with, without question. As my last week approached, I was feeling sad. I was already missing the Clubhouse.

While in my office cleaning things out on my last Monday morning of work there, I received a phone call from the receptionist at the Clubhouse that there were two people at the reception desk who wanted to meet with me. This brought back a memory of the last time I had received a call that two people wanted to meet with me at the reception area. That had been well over a year ago.

When I got to the reception area that time, there were two women dressed like the Keystone Cops standing by the reception desk. Donning blue uniforms with big shiny brass buttons on a double-breasted coat, they had stuffed the coat so that they had little paunchy bellies. Bowler caps and fake mustaches finished off the look. The cops made a big show of being there to arrest me for various "crimes" as they loudly accused me of being nice and a good boss. They took out a pair of fuzzy red handcuffs to put around my wrists much to the amusement of staff and members. The Keystone Cops led me out of the Clubhouse and put me into their "cop car" which happened to be this incredible limousine. That was the one and only time I have ever been in such a fancy vehicle. They even offered me a soft drink and snacks on the ride to "jail." The jail was at a popular car dealership. They had a makeshift jail with fake bars all around a designated area. There were four or five other people in the jail looking through their rolodexes and lists of phone numbers. They were busily making phone calls asking for donations to make their "bail."

Apparently, this arrest was part of a fundraiser for a local charity. I was the only one who had no idea about the "arrest" and the fundraiser. I made one call to the Clubhouse. As a continuation of their joke on me, they denied they even knew me stating that their director (me) had just been arrested and incarcerated. Three or four members and staff showed up within a half hour with a loaf of bread and a file folder telling me they had come to break me out of jail. They were truly having a good laugh about this. They had taken up a collection and were able to make my bail. I was freed in just a little more than an hour. It is a memory I will treasure not only because of how effectively they all pulled off the stunt, but also because in reality, they were letting me know that they really cared about and appreciated me. We had such a good laugh over the entire experience.

On that last Monday morning of work at the Clubhouse, I wondered what they were up to this time as I made it over to the reception area. There was a heavy feeling of stress that almost stopped me in my tracks as I entered that part of the building. Waiting for me at the reception desk were two men dressed in suit coats with a very official look to them. They introduced themselves stating they were detectives from the city police station. They asked if there was somewhere we could meet in private. I took them up to my office. They looked so serious that even before I knew why they were there, I had a dreadful feeling in the pit of my stomach.

They explained that something tragic had happened Saturday night and a body had been found floating in the river early Sunday morning. There was no identification on the body and they were unable to identify it. One of the beat policemen at the police station stated that he recognized the person but did not know their name. He explained that he often saw the person hanging around our Clubhouse. The detectives asked if they could show me some photographs of the body to help them determine who it was.

I hesitated and almost said no. I wasn't sure if I could handle that responsibility. However, I heard the word okay come out of my mouth. One of the detectives reached into the inside pocket of his jacket taking out an envelope. He withdrew a series of photographs. They were laid across my desk for me to see them in their entirety. The photos were grotesque and showed a bloated and bruised body.

"Oh no!" I blurted out. "I know who that is. It's Tom. He is a member here. What happened???"

As I became tearful the detective quickly reassembled the photos and placed them back in the envelope and into his inside jacket pocket. "We are so sorry for your loss," the other detective responded to my obvious hurt and shock. "We don't know what happened," he said. "It could have been suicide or an accident or an attack that led to murder. We just don't know right now. But we will do everything we can to find out."

He shared that there was evidence of some kind of a struggle on the bridge closest to the Clubhouse. Some of Tom's clothing was strewn on the sidewalk with other personal items, but nothing that identified who the body was. They surmised that was where Tom had fallen into the river, either on his own or following a struggle with other persons. "Something happened on that bridge," the detective concluded.

He asked if he could have a list of Tom's contacts. They wanted to inform a family member about the death. I shared what we had on Tom. Part of being a member is leaving us with the number of an emergency contact person. The detectives took the contact information for Tom's mother. They questioned me about Tom. They wanted to know if I had noticed anything unusual about Tom and his behavior in the past few weeks. In particular, they asked if he seemed more depressed or out of sorts than usual.

A tornado of memories, thoughts, and emotions swirled around and began to flood my brain when those questions were asked. There was so much going on for Tom, especially within the last year. Where do I even begin to answer those questions?

I met Tom over two years prior to this conversation. He was referred to the Clubhouse by his state social worker. He had been hospitalized for depression and anxiety. At that time, he received a diagnosis of major depressive disorder and anxiety disorder. He and his social worker determined that involvement at the Clubhouse would be helpful for him. Tom was in his mid to late twenties. He told me he had always felt like an imposter when it came to his life.

School, socializing, and making friends were always challenging for Tom. He became depressed because he could not determine where he fit in. However, Tom had a warm personality. At the Clubhouse he was easy to be around and he was so kind to all of the other members.

Tom became a regular and involved member. What a delightful and caring person he was. When it came to choosing what area of the Clubhouse he wanted to work in, he chose the kitchen. He joked that it had a lot to do with the fact that he really liked to eat. However, he chose it because he liked to cook and enjoyed serving meals to people. He got so much enjoyment and satisfaction when a member would pay a compliment to the chefs. He was especially delighted when somebody absolutely loved their meal. That was what came across immediately when you met Tom. He had a servant's heart. He smiled and laughed almost all the time. He had a gentleness and genuineness about him that endeared him to all of us.

About a year after he began coming to the Clubhouse, he started coming in wearing a wig and women's clothing. He shared with the members at one of our daily meetings that he wanted to be addressed as "Sheila." So, we did. Sheila continued to participate at the Clubhouse, working in the kitchen. However, in the past few months she'd started to participate less in our social activities. She also cut back on how many days of the week she came. When I noticed that Sheila was less present, I checked with staff, inquiring if they had any information regarding Sheila's change in participation. I was concerned that she was uncomfortable about being at the Clubhouse. Her supervisor in the kitchen shared that she hadn't noticed that. It seemed that she was still the delightful and enjoyable person she had always been. Other members appeared to be supportive and accepting of her and nothing in her behavior while she was at the Clubhouse indicated that anything was wrong.

I filled in the detectives on what was going on for Tom, whom we had come to know as Sheila. It was important to inform them of her transition. While it seemed that she was comfortable at the Clubhouse, many of us worried that there would be some people in the city who would not understand. Quite honestly, there was much that we, at the Clubhouse, did not understand about what Sheila was going through. There were times she was guarded about the changes that were happening in her life. Perhaps she was also trying to figure out her own feelings about what she was experiencing. Because we had come to love and appreciate her, we accepted her as she was. We suspected that she had found other places where she also felt welcomed. We knew that she had friends in the LGBTQ community and was spending more time with them. That being said, we were fortunate enough to know that it is the same spirit that gave Sheila her spark and Tom his gentleness. We enjoyed coming to know and have Sheila as a part of our small community.

The detectives shared that the body they found in the river was a male wearing women's clothing. They had also witnessed the disrespect for members of the LGBTQ community within the city that was going on as she transitioned from Tom to Sheila. They were concerned that there may have been some foul play. I shared with them that we worried about that for Sheila as well. We talked about how judgmental and cruel some people can be when it comes to what Sheila was experiencing. The detectives shared that the LGBTQ community was a very vulnerable group and there had been a number of assaults in the city on their community. While I was not surprised to hear that, Sheila had never shared with us anything related to being harmed or accosted.

The detectives left after they had the information for which they had come. I stayed up in my office for a bit of time afterwards trying to process what I had just experienced. Emotional numbness took over as I sat there unable to move. It was not because I didn't feel anything but because I was feeling too much. It was overwhelming and I couldn't sort through it. It didn't make any sense that Sheila would have committed suicide and I did not want to think that Sheila had been murdered. Both scenarios were too awful.

I knew that the detectives left without saying a word to anyone else. I knew that our staff and members would be left confused and concerned because of their appearance. It was time to call the receptionist and ask her to send the staff to my office for a short meeting.

They entered my office quietly and with much confusion and concern on their faces. We all were in shock and disbelief as I shared what I could about what the detectives had told me about Sheila.

We cried and we comforted each other. None of us could accept that Sheila would have killed herself. Considering that Sheila could have been murdered was horrifying. We processed this as best we could that Monday morning. How were we going to share this news with our members? How could we be a support for Sheila's family? Somehow, decisions and plans were made. Two of us were going to meet Sheila's mother as soon as we could that day. We also decided that we would take as many people as we could to whatever funeral services were planned for her.

Sheila's primary supervisor shared the news with the members at our daily meeting. More tears were shed and shock expressed.

None of us wanted to believe something so awful had happened to someone we cared about so dearly.

I was fortunate to meet Sheila's mother on that fateful Monday. I had never met her before, but as soon as I did, I saw Sheila in her. I was taken aback at how much mother and child looked so much alike in facial features and body type. They were both sweet and emotional. It was wonderful to meet her. We cried and shared stories of her sweet loving child. We also shared laughter about the many enjoyable characteristics of her delightful son. She expressed her gratitude that Tom had such caring people in his life. She referred to him as Tom, not because she did not accept what was happening for Tom, but mainly because that is how she had known him for so much of his life. She did say often that she loved him no matter what.

When we returned to the Clubhouse a number of us, staff and members, talked about how we recognized that Sheila was coming to terms with who she felt she really was inside. Sharing this reality with others must have been so difficult for her. We suspected that she was spending more time with others who were experiencing what she was. Hopefully, she did find others who could help her to understand and accept herself better. However, in placing herself within that community, we feared she put herself at risk. The detectives indicated their fear was that someone had taken it upon themselves to let her know that her current behaviors and associations would not be tolerated. The detectives knew of others in that community who had been accosted and assaulted. They, and I, feared the worst had happened.

"Something happened on that bridge." That phrase the detective shared kept circling through my mind. It was simply incongruous that something so awful, something so divisive would happen on that bridge. The bridge the detective had mentioned was so familiar to me and to everyone else at the Clubhouse. I crossed that bridge every day to get back and forth from work. That bridge connected one side of the city with the other. The bridge lay over that powerful and beautiful river. Some days the river was as quiet as a church, other days that river churned and complained and had a menacing presence. Day after day, that bridge stood its ground and provided passage, safety, and assurance. Bridges are about what connects us. Bridges unite two separate shores. They literally cross troubled waters to join differing sides. How utterly cruel that the demise of Sheila would be on that beautiful bridge.

When thinking about what had happened to Sheila, the question of why just would not go away. Did what happened to Sheila have to do with intolerance and divisiveness? For all of history, we humans have found any number of reasons to reject, vilify, and eliminate people who do not fit into whatever norms a society feels must be enforced. Prejudice, bigotry, and hatefulness are part of the history of so many societies and communities. I chose to work with people who I knew are marginalized because of their mental illnesses and life challenges. I knew that I would be working with people that many others would not understand. In fact, many of the people with whom I worked over the years had to endure much fear and misunderstanding from many intolerant and ignorant people and communities where they lived.

It is not just ignorance that leads to hateful and intolerant beliefs and judgements. It is a mindset where some would "other" people whom they do not understand. It is a mindset where their judgement leads to decisions that "those people" are evil and unfit for society. Because of that label, it is determined that we can jail them, institutionalize them, put them in concentration camps or kill them. That mindset tells people who fear "the other" that if something isn't done to remove those "evil people" from society they will poison and ruin our world.

What I know from my belief system is that all people are valuable and beloved children of the God who is love. Harsh judgements, selfishness, greed, and intolerance have nothing to do with a faith that is based on a loving God. When I recognize those unjust attitudes and the behaviors associated with those attitudes in me. I seek out help from God, and from other believers, to change them. This is what I have come to know about my faith. That is why I stay connected with other believers who can remind me and help me to be a better person, a more tolerant person, a more loving person. I fall short of this every day, multiple times a day. I need to make time all day, every day, to remind myself to whom I belong. I belong to a God who is all about love.

I do understand that many persons of faith are exactly those who most demonstrate bigotry and hatefulness towards others. Thoughts, beliefs, and attitudes that reflect hatefulness, misunderstanding, and intolerance from a religious tradition seem contradictory to me. It is more than unfortunate that these attitudes become part of an institutional response that is passed down from generation to generation. Hatefulness and intolerance, even though they are disguised as morality, are really what can poison an innocent child or person who naturally knows that all people have value.

In reality, this chosen field of mine meant that I would encounter many clients over the years who did die for a number of reasons. Some of the clients I worked with did commit suicide. Some of them passed away from natural causes. A number of people I worked with died from drug overdoses. Sheila is the only person I worked with over the decades that might have been murdered, that most likely was murdered. That is just horrible. Thirty-two years after her death, I am still horrified that a human being thought they had the right to kill another human being just because they judged her as a threat, a sin, an evil. Shame on them. She was so young. She was so loved and so loving. She was a truly remarkable person.

That last week I was at the Clubhouse was difficult and emotional. The final thing I did in that last week was go to the funeral on Friday. It was a sad and moving experience. Many of us were there and said our goodbyes and thank yous to Sheila for her bravery, her honesty, and her care and love for all of us.

Sheila challenged me to be brave and to be an advocate whenever I could for those who are marginalized and "othered." The race and culture we are born into, the color of our skin, mental illness, addiction, sexual orientation; none of these are a choice and are not an indication of moral weakness. They are not evil and they will not poison our society. Hatefulness is chosen.

Mindsets that vilify people who are not evil are poisonous. That is the poison that creates divisiveness and hostility. Wouldn't it be better if we worked on understanding, tolerance, and building bridges instead of creating obstacles?

CHAPTER 4

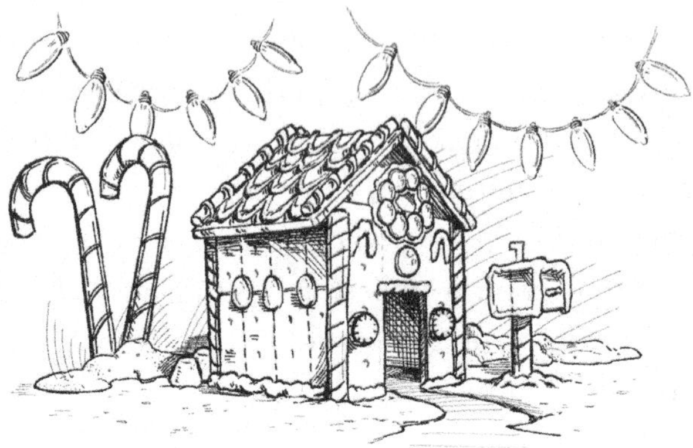

Emotional Superglue

Because there is so much variety in mental health work and providing psychotherapy, I was a licensed mental health counselor for a few years before I started doing mainly office-based counseling. This involves meeting with an individual client in a private office for counseling based on a client's stated needs and concerns. The intensity of relationships developed in this setting is difficult to describe. The client who comes in for psychotherapy is utterly exposed as they share their vulnerability in asking for help because something has overwhelmed them, interrupted their daily lives and made things a bit too difficult to manage on their own. My exposure as a therapist was also an issue. Would I be helpful? Did I really have the ability to listen well enough, problem solve effectively enough, and be present and strong enough to help a client help themselves?

What I began to learn as I developed as a psychotherapist was that it would be the clients who would help me the most to understand what strength is and what it means to be enough. One of the clients who was particularly helpful to me in learning this lesson was Anne.

A thin, attractive woman in her mid to late fifties, Anne came to her first appointment with one issue: she wanted to be able to take the elevator to pick up her mail at the senior housing complex where she had recently moved. She thought that if she could get that handled, she would be fine. She explained her dilemma: "I am having trouble leaving my apartment. I don't know what to say if someone talks to me. I wait for days before I go pick up my mail. You can't believe how many people hang out by the mailboxes."

Going to pick up her mail took strenuous emotional effort. Some days she would spend an hour or more giving herself a pep talk just to get out of her apartment. She just could not stomach taking the elevator if there were other people in the elevator with her. In fact, most days Anne would wait until the middle of the night and sneak down at 2:00 a.m. to avoid running into people. She was particularly uncomfortable about going to the mailboxes because there was always someone in that area getting mail or talking with neighbors in the building. There were more people at the mailboxes than any other place at the senior living complex.

So, that is where we started. We focused on getting her to the mailboxes to get her mail. Anne had moved into the high-rise building in her native city about three or four months before she started seeing me for therapy. Up until her move to the complex, she had spent her entire life in her family home. She had stayed behind as her siblings got married or joined the military and moved away to live their own adult lives. She worked out of the home for a while doing a factory job. Her father passed away when Anne was in her late thirties. Being devoted to her mother, Anne remained in the home to look after her. Over the years as her mother needed more care, Anne gave up her factory job. She looked after her mother for many years. Her mother passed away about a year ago. As such, the family home was sold and Anne had to move.

Initially, we focused on managing anxiety and trying out some behavioral changes to help her to get out of her apartment and to the mailboxes. Counseling is always a better experience when clients are motivated. Anne was that kind of a client. Although she was very anxious and unsure of herself, she wanted to have a better life experience. She was open and curious about approaches that could help with her anxiety. She wanted to know more about her current emotions that sometimes worsened her behaviors. She wanted to learn how to understand her emotions and make changes to behaviors that were holding her back. So, she made some adjustments and, lo and behold, getting into and out of the elevator and to the mailboxes became easier for her.

Anne presented as someone "uncomplicated." Early in counseling, she would often say, "I have never been a difficult person. I get along with everyone." Family was often a topic during our sessions. Family is where she had put most of her time and emotional energy throughout her life. While Anne seemed to be a fairly uncomplicated person, it seemed that her family and upbringing were anything but. Being the second youngest of nine siblings is in itself complicated. Eleven people living in the same space can be chaotic. That's eleven different personalities, needs, interests, habits, volumes, and body sizes. She talked about her family with fondness, but I suspected that there was much more to the story.

Anne discovered that she really liked to talk. She had not known that about herself because she never really had a chance to talk. We made a connection and she was pleasantly surprised that I was genuinely interested in her and wanted to know about her and her stories. She had lots of stories. As she made progress and opened up more about herself and her life, the stories of family difficulties and abuse were shared. It was difficult for Anne to share about family problems. She needed to test me to determine if it was safe or not. When she determined it was safe the stories were shared. With very little eye contact and a soft voice she shared stories about her father's alcohol abuse. Her father had an explosive drunken temper. When intoxicated he would become loud and obnoxious as he shouted aggressive and cruel put-downs to his sons. He would ignore and disrespect his wife, whom Anne adored. Her father was not often physically abusive, but when he was, it would scare her terribly. These episodes left little Anne a very anxious child.

One day Anne came to our therapy appointment with a book that she had just bought at Buck-a-Book in downtown Providence. "Look what I found at Buck-a-Book! It has all these great projects and I thought we could go through them together." Anne was unusually excited about this find and her enthusiasm was quite infectious.

"Absolutely! What a great idea. Where would you like to start?"

"We can start at the beginning," she enthused, sounding like a happy excited child as she opened the book to the first few pages. The book was *A Workbook for Healing Adult Children of Alcoholics* by Patty McConnell.

A few days later I went to Buck-a-Book to purchase my own copy. As I familiarized myself with the book, it reminded me of my job back in Lynn, Massachusetts at CHAOS. It seemed to echo the expressive arts approach that we used regularly in that treatment setting. I did most of the book's exercises on my own before doing them in the sessions with Anne. That way I could have a bit of an understanding of what it would be like for her.

At her next appointment, we started at the beginning. However, we made it our own. Exercises were adjusted to fit Anne and her personality, strengths, and interests.

One of the early exercises was to draw pictures of the family home and the people in that home. Anne had an idea of how she wanted to do it. It was not exactly how the book laid it out and I encouraged her to do it her way.

At the next session, an enthusiastic and proud Anne presented her drawing. She had put much thought into the project. The drawing was wonderful! It was colorful and well sketched out on a small white poster board. Displayed in the drawing was a home that had three levels. It opened up to the viewer as if you were looking into a dollhouse. She carefully pointed out what was in her drawing. She pointed out each room and its significance, including what and who was in each room. She presented each family member and the reason she had drawn them in the room they were in. As she shared about who was in each room and why, more important stories about Anne's life were revealed. There was much back-and-forth as she shared her drawing and welcomed my questions and comments. After she was done describing her family home, I looked at her and asked as benignly as I could, "Where are you?"

She carefully looked at her drawing and then burst into tears. "I don't know," she choked out. Anne had not put herself into the drawing of her family home.

I asked her gently, "If you were to draw yourself into the drawing, where would you be?"

"Under the bed," she cried.

As difficult as it was, Anne talked about her not being in the drawing and about how painful that felt. She believed that she needed to hide in order to feel safe in her home. With very little eye contact as tears streamed down her face, she cried that she did not want to be seen, although that was not at all true. She just didn't know if it was safe to be seen. For many years she had been wondering and perhaps believing that no one in the family really wanted to see her, to know her, or to acknowledge her.

This began the real work of her counseling experience. Did she really want to take the risk of being seen and known? Did she even know who she really was? Wouldn't it just be easier and safer if she stayed under her "emotional bed?"

Thankfully, Anne kept coming for her sessions. We continued working with the workbook. It was so helpful because the next few chapters provided opportunities to use more expressive arts—writing, poetry, and drawing—to address the hurts that were part of her upbringing. She worked on beliefs, the roles she assumed from being part of a dysfunctional family and the self-sabotage that is born from that upbringing.

When we got to the chapters on healing, she was no longer hiding under that emotional bed. Her life began to reflect a new confidence and determination. She made friends with a neighbor and even started going to bingo games at the housing complex with her. It was fascinating to witness her coming into her own, feeling happy and strong about being herself and letting other people know who she was.

When she would come into a session and share a new experience, I would tease her a bit and say "Who are you??" Remarkably, she would laugh and totally enjoy being seen just for who she was.

Home became a recurring theme for our counseling sessions after that family home drawing. We had many conversations about the adult responsibility to become your own home and to feel at home in your own skin no matter where you live. She loved coming up with metaphors of her own about being home and making the world her home, whether others saw her or not.

In early December, Anne arrived at a session stating that she was going to make herself a gingerbread house for Christmas. She had always wanted to do that and this was the year she would make one. I made her promise to take a picture of her house and bring it into a session. A week before Christmas, she came in for her session with a very large bag and a very mischievous smile on her face.

"I have something for you," she said as she pulled out a gingerbread house on a small wooden platform.

"It's a gingerbread house!" I exclaimed. "It's just beautiful!"

"I made it for you," she said excitedly. "You can have it."

I teared up as I responded, "It looks delicious!"

"You can't eat it!" she replied immediately. "I had some trouble keeping the walls up with the icing, so I used some superglue. And

I also used superglue to keep the gumdrops on and some of the M&Ms and peppermints too. Don't eat it."

She explained that getting the icing to the exact consistency needed to keep the gingerbread together and the candies to stay in place was much harder than she had expected. So, she came up with the superglue solution. Once the gingerbread stayed together with the superglue, she could then add the icing and the decorations. I complimented her on her problem-solving skills, because clearly, she got the desired result. It was a completed, nicely decorated gingerbread house. She was so proud of her creation.

As asked, she had a picture of the house she made for herself that we viewed together on her cell phone. She also showed me pictures of the gingerbread houses she made for her friend at the housing complex and the ones she made for her sisters. She really got into making gingerbread houses that Christmas season!

It wasn't long after that Anne decided to end her counseling. She had come such a long way. I sent her off knowing that she would be just fine.

I am so grateful to Anne for all the things I learned from her. She introduced me to that great workbook. This was a resource that was later used with many other clients because it was extremely effective. She reminded me that using creativity is an important part of our healing and it is important to find ways to include that while doing therapy with clients. I found that making time for my own creative interests was going to benefit me in my work as a therapist as well. Especially when I felt that I was getting overwhelmed, or burnt out, that was a reminder to make time for my own creative interests. I needed to sit at the piano for a bit, join a choir, or do some sewing, knitting, or handwork. Leave it to Anne—I also developed a new appreciation for gingerbread houses.

I began to reflect on the many problem-solving skills that Anne developed as she worked through the pain, hurt, and anxiety she had been carrying for so long. It seemed to me that Anne developed her own "emotional superglue" to work through the difficulties of her own life. She became stronger and more resilient as she learned not only about the hurts of life but also about the strengths she always had inside of her. Once she did find those inner strengths, look out world, because she was determined to make the world her home.

Don't we all have times where we need a bit of emotional superglue to help keep us from falling apart? Sometimes the emotional icing that we are taught to develop from our family systems is just not strong enough. We find ourselves falling apart, hiding under our own emotional beds because we just don't feel strong enough to be seen. Or we don't know any other ways to keep ourselves safe. Developing resilience for the tough things in life is our emotional superglue.

I am always amazed at how God uses such ordinary moments to remind us of important life lessons. For instance, when I was in the process of writing this story, I received a fortune cookie that said, "To be resilient is to bounce back from life's challenges with strength." How did God or whatever loving presence is looking out for me know that I needed to get that fortune? It helped me to name what I knew had happened with Anne. In her case, she needed to find and develop resiliency where there may have been little. She needed to learn to push back her fear to find out how strong she actually was.

This is what I have come to know. We don't need to go looking for ways to develop resilience. Our own lives will do that for us on a regular basis. Challenges, hurts, disappointments, consequential mistakes are part of everyone's life. The resilience we tap into within ourselves will help determine how we manage our way through those most difficult life experiences. I think of my own difficult challenges: not being able to have children, going through a divorce, getting cancer. While it felt that I was falling apart in those moments, I didn't. I reached in and I reached out to find my own emotional superglue. What I found was the grace and love of God, the caring and support of family and friends, and an inner strength that was always a part of me, though there were times I forgot to look for it and make use of it. With my beliefs and the support of those around me, and my inner resilience, the walls did not come tumbling down. In fact, those experiences helped me to be a better and stronger person.

Whether it is finding a book at the discount bookstore, drawing a picture, glueing together a gingerbread house, or opening up a fortune cookie, life will always present us with experiences and people that remind us to be grateful for our strengths. Because of what I learned from Anne, I have more awareness of my own resilience, fortitude, and "emotional superglue."

CHAPTER 5

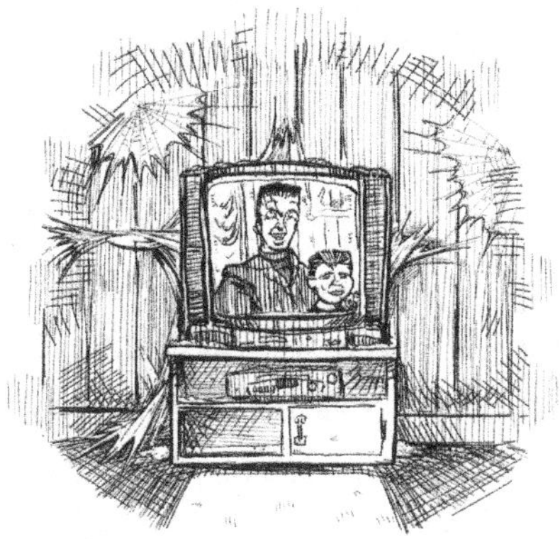

Removing Cobwebs

Working in community mental health was both a gift and a challenge. There were hundreds of lessons I learned from clients over the years. Some of them, actually most of them, were a bit hard taught. I learned those lessons because I was doing something that was not at all helpful. But the kindness and honesty of the clients I worked with provided me with what I most needed to learn. The beauty of lessons learned is that they continue to teach me long after the initial experience.

I was doing home visits at the time, supporting adults with chronic and persistent mental illness in their efforts to live independently in their own homes and apartments. I was part of a community support team for clients who were dealing with challenging personal situations, working as the master's level clinician.

We saw Mary daily at her apartment in a public housing project. In her mid-thirties, she was such a sweet, quiet, and dutiful person. Every morning, she opened her door for us, let us into her kitchen, and would visit with us for a few minutes. Mary had a thought disorder including hallucinations and delusions, and from time to time she would become paranoid and disturbed. She had a number of hospitalizations over the years and was diagnosed with paranoid schizophrenia.

One of our jobs was to watch Mary take her morning medication in an attempt to assure that for the most part her mental health symptoms would not interfere in her daily life. One of the members of our home visiting team was also selected to offer more intensive support and was tasked to work as her primary caseworker. That staff member's job was to help her to identify and work on needs and goals. In other words—the treatment plan. I became the person to assist Mary with this task.

Ideally, we preferred that clients identify their own needs and set goals that were their own, but in all honesty, it wasn't that easy for Mary to work on this. So, I did what I could to address what was needed and come up with ideas on how our team could help her to help herself.

Our supervisors and agency leadership presented that the treatment plan was akin to a medical doctor writing a patient a prescription. Somehow, we needed to justify the work we were doing and show that we addressed needs, identified goals, and created a plan to meet those goals. Our funding sources, mostly the state, required that each client have a treatment plan. The state also had particular suggestions as to what should be a part of a client's plan. We had to put in the goal of seeing a psychiatrist and following a psychiatrist's medical plan—i.e., taking medication to help control psychiatric symptoms and avoid hospitalizations. There needed to be goals about medical needs and addressing housing concerns as well as social and vocational opportunities. So, getting those needs identified and coming up with plans to address those needs was something that had to get done. That was one of the major expectations of a client's primary caseworker's job.

Now Mary's apartment was a bit of a mess. It was dingy, dark and gray. As soon as you entered the apartment you would notice cobwebs in the corners of the ceiling and floors, and stretching from her furniture to the wall. There were cobwebs and dust everywhere. It was not a very pleasant place to visit—never mind actually living within that space. So naturally, working on keeping a clean apartment was identified as a need and a goal. But that really was not Mary's goal. She was not at all interested in cleaning her apartment "thank you very much." She appeared to be resisting this goal in particular, so it seemed to me. I thought she was being difficult, until I stumbled upon a truth that changed everything.

The TV was always on in Mary's apartment when the team would come for our visits. Since I spent more time with her than other staff, I would sit and talk with her and watch a little TV once in a while. One day, as we sat together by her TV, I asked her if she had a favorite TV show. She immediately brightened up and responded "I love *The Munsters*!" She proceeded to talk excitedly about how she loved the show, the characters in the show, and how they made her laugh. She ended with the statement "I like that show so much I decorated my apartment to look just like their house."

And so she had. "Mary, Mary quite contrary" was not contrary at all. She was inspired by her favorite TV show is all. *The Munsters* was a popular TV show in the 1960s featuring a cast of characters who made up a benign monster family who lived in the suburbs. The show included a Frankenstein father named Herman, his vampire wife Lily, and their werewolf son Eddie, along with a few others. They lived in a scary house on the hill, complete with bats in the belfry and plenty of cobwebs and dust and dinginess within and without. Mary took it upon herself to make her own apartment reflect what she saw on her favorite TV show. It must have taken quite a bit of commitment on her part to get to the state of dreariness and Munster-like appeal she actually did achieve.

Luckily, I did respond with some positivity and congratulated her on how well she did achieve the look of the Munsters' home. I must admit that while I was inwardly laughing at how all of us had missed her efforts and creativity, I was also embarrassed by my judgmentalness. It was impressive that she had been resisting cleaning her apartment because, for her, it was exactly as she wanted it to be. I decided to not focus on the cleaning of her apartment (so much) until she was ready.

We continued to bond as she became more talkative and engaging. I decided to explore other TV shows she liked. After all, *The Munsters* had not made a new episode in decades and was just in reruns as Mary pointed out.

Mary is Hispanic and she really enjoyed the novellas from Mexico and South America. We made a plan for me to use one of my support visits to watch her favorite novella together. I don't remember the name of the show but it was in Spanish and quite dramatic. This novella was about people in a city setting—I think Mexico City. Her favorite character had a beautiful apartment in a high-rise apartment building. We talked about her reaction to the novella. She loved the drama, including the fights and betrayals and cliff-hangers. She was lukewarm about the romance. I asked if she could ever see herself living in an apartment like her favorite character. She took some time to consider her answer. She glanced around at her cobweb infested dingy apartment and answered, "Yes. I would like that."

We took our time as she continued to contemplate changing her apartment decor. We talked about what she envisioned—colors, patterns (florals were quite popular in that novella). We made a plan and she started to save her money. We set a date to clear out the cobwebs, dust the furniture, shake out the rugs, and wash the windows. This took some time and when the apartment was as clean as she wanted it to be and enough money had been saved, we went shopping.

She got all dressed up and even put a little make-up on for the trip to the discount store where she would buy curtains and bedding, kitchen placemats, and some doilies. We hauled everything into the apartment. She was exhausted, but excited at the same time. We reviewed the importance of going at her own pace knowing there was no rush on this.

A few days later I stopped by. Mary opened the door smiling, proudly showing off her kitchen placemats set up in a clean kitchen. The bedroom had also been cleaned and decorated with her new purchases. It was lovely. We put up the curtains in her living room and put out the doilies on the living room side tables. Her apartment makeover was complete.

She was delighted. This experience even led to a change in her own appearance. The Lily Munster wardrobe she previously sported consisted of mainly gray and black shirts and pants and an occasional black skirt and blouse. Tall and slender with shoulder-length black, thick, and curly hair, the colorful pants and shirts she now wore made her look like a completely different person.

It was remarkable how this change of decor and outfits made such a difference. Mary had worked on and met a goal that was her own goal. It was her own vision. How gratifying to see how committed she was to updating her apartment and keeping it as clean as she could.

Now, the fact remains that Mary continued to have symptoms of her mental illness. She still heard voices and experienced delusions and paranoia. Some days were harder than others and her apartment never was very clean or perfectly kept. But that was all okay.

She taught me a valuable lesson. Our lives are our own. I had fallen into the trap of thinking that I knew more about her than she did. I made my agenda more important than her. My internal vision was marred by my own inner cobwebs and dingy emotional windows. I didn't realize how much I had become overly influenced by the pressure and expectation to meet the larger institutional requirements. My focus got blurred. When something is not clear emotionally it is hard to see through to a clearer and more just path. But God is good and through God's grace one day I stumbled upon a good question: "Do you have a favorite TV show?" That is what made the difference—a simple, unexpected question.

As we worked on her plan to remove the cobwebs, clean the windows, and sweep out the dust, I am sure that both of us were cleaning out our own dingy hearts and minds, allowing a bit of time for clearer vision. In particular, I was learning to suspend judgment and make room for curiosity and connection. Asking questions is 100 percent a part of a therapist's job. What has stayed with me is the importance of being more mindful about asking good questions. What I learned especially from that experience is that clients matter more than institutions. Of course, I knew that in my mind, but I needed to learn it as part of building a healthy, respectful relationship with clients. Certainly, connecting with clients to help them have a better life experience is why I pursued this work.

Mary absolutely taught me how to value that experience more than I had been. I learned in a most unexpected way that questions really do matter.

CHAPTER 6

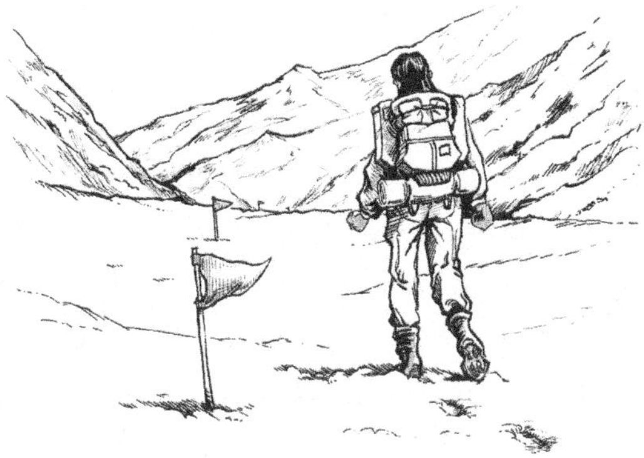

To the Mall

Much of what I learned and trained for in graduate school anticipated that I would be working in an office setting with individuals, groups, couples, or families focusing on some form of talk therapy. That has been the traditional form of psychotherapy for decades and decades. For me, I thoroughly enjoyed therapy that happened outside of an office setting. I suppose it is because most of my early experience and training involved working with people with severe and persistent mental illness. Office-based counseling in a small office sitting face-to-face was not usually the most effective way to reach and connect with people who had chronic and persistent mental illness. If someone is experiencing delusions, or hallucinations on a regular basis, having a reality-based conversation in a small room with someone looking at you in many cases can worsen symptoms and increase feelings of paranoia. If someone is experiencing mania, sitting still in an office is also very challenging, if not impossible. Someone in a manic episode is not going to show up for a therapy appointment. Likewise for persons with severe depression; getting to any appointment, or even out of the house, takes strenuous effort. So, from the beginning, I was naturally led to think out of the box when doing psychotherapy with a person who was struggling with a severe mental illness.

One of the things I liked best about being the master level clinician on our mobile treatment team was finding creative approaches in providing individual therapy with each client. The ideas that surfaced mostly came from the clients themselves. Nadia was referred for counseling by her psychiatrist and primary caseworker with concerns that while Nadia had made some progress since her last hospitalization, she was slipping back into isolative behaviors and negativity. Although we had a challenging beginning, what Nadia and I figured out together seemed to make a positive and helpful difference for her.

Nadia was born and raised in Eastern Europe. She moved to the United States with her two young children in the 1990s when things in that part of the world were very unstable. She came to a country where she could barely speak the language and everything was unfamiliar—the streets, the housing, the food, the people and the pace of life. She did her best to work at adjusting to all the changes. However, by the end of her first year here she was not doing well at all.

She felt weak and incompetent as she witnessed her two children adjust to the move so much quicker than she. They learned English and were doing well in school. They were making friends and becoming Americanized. Not so with Nadia. Depending on her children to translate at appointments or with their teachers at school conferences was an embarrassment. Not being able to help her children with their homework or understand their school schedules or bus routes was an ultimate humiliation. She believed she was failing her children and questioned if she were failing as a person.

Nadia became severely depressed as she felt more overwhelmed with the demands of life in this newly adopted country. In addition to having so much difficulty getting herself involved in her daily life, she also developed a bit of a psychotic response to her depression. She said and did bizarre things that freaked out her family. She stopped allowing her children to leave the home. She blocked off the door to her porch fearing that someone was going to climb up to her second-story apartment and steal her children. Her children would see her mumbling to herself as she stopped her own self-care of bathing and changing her clothes. One of her sisters had immigrated to the United States before her and was able to move to Rhode Island to help her and her family. Her sister also noticed and became extremely concerned about Nadia's failing mental health. Even with that assistance, Nadia continued to deteriorate and was admitted to a psychiatric hospital. She was a single parent with two young school-age children and the state's Department of Children, Youth and Families became involved as her ability to parent was tested and questioned. Her children were removed from her care as a result of the hospitalization and went to stay with their aunt.

She was devastated when her children were removed. Our team was brought in to help provide more intensive treatment and support as part of her hospital discharge plan. We were able to meet with her in her home daily. She and her psychiatrist found a medication regimen that was helpful. Thankfully, regular visits with her children began and they would come for supper a few times a week. Slowly her debilitating depression was lessening.

Even with daily contact and support from our team and her sister, Nadia was still having trouble getting out of her apartment. A very religious person, she wanted to become more active in a nearby church as a way to help decrease the isolation. Feelings of insignificance and inferiority were getting in the way of her participation in church. Our team hoped that we could help minimize and eliminate the feelings of guilt and sinfulness she was adding to the baggage of her perceived feeling of failure because she wasn't getting to church.

Nadia was referred to meet with me for some psychotherapy to work on the depression, anxiety, and self-esteem issues that were blocking some of her forward progress. Our first appointment happened in her apartment. As I entered into a darkened home with curtains and shades drawn, my eyes had to adjust to the only real light in the apartment that was coming from her television.

She was plopped on the couch blankly staring at the TV screen dressed in sweatpants and a wrinkled shirt. Slouching on the couch made her already overweight body look bloated and unhealthy. Her short light brown hair was unkempt and unclean, and an unfinished breakfast lay on the floor near the couch. Allowing me to enter the apartment, she did not look at me and barely acknowledged my presence. Reluctantly, she agreed to turn off the TV. She would not move into the kitchen area to sit and talk at her table where there was a little more light. So, we talked for a bit in her darkened living room. I explained why I was there, stating that her psychiatrist asked me to come and offer her some therapy, hoping that counseling could help her to continue and build on the progress she had recently made following her hospitalization.

She was not interested in much of what I presented about talk therapy. "I don't like to talk. I don't talk English good," was her mantra that day. By this time, Nadia had been in the US for a few years. While Nadia's English was not that good, it was certainly good enough for us to do some basic therapy and I knew that she knew that, but I did not refute her. We did have some conversation about things that she used to like to do. The only time she almost smiled involved talking about how she used to enjoy shopping and getting things for her children. However, she was no longer in a financial position to do that. She was not working and her social security income barely covered her monthly bills. I have to be honest, that first appointment didn't go so well. All that first appointment did was remind her of another way she was failing her children and she felt even worse. Needless to say, we did not make a good connection with each other that day.

The next time we met was at the office. With some encouragement from her psychiatrist and primary caseworker she had agreed to meet with me one more time. Actually, she was coming in to meet with her psychiatrist. Otherwise, I would not have had the benefit of one more attempt to start some counseling. After she met with him, she sat down with me for a short time. It seemed that she harbored a little crush on the psychiatrist because she always came into the office well dressed and a bit more animated. I decided to start there, letting her talk about what she liked about him. Before me was a Nadia that looked and sounded a bit like a high school girl in puppy love. "I like him much." With a shy smile she described how handsome he was and how nice he was to her.

"He is very easy to like," I responded. I commented on how nice she looked that day. Blushing and appreciative of the compliment, she shared that her daughter had let her borrow some of her make-up. There followed much talk about her daughter's trips to the Providence Place Mall where she had gotten some free samples at the make-up counter at Nordstrom's. I revisited our conversation about shopping. I described how a lot of people go to the mall not to buy things but just to window-shop. I told her how my mother and aunts had outings to the mall at least once a week just to walk around, look, browse, and spend time together. Often, they didn't buy anything at all. She was fascinated by that. Visiting the Providence Mall was of great interest to her. Finding a connection, we were able to work on a plan to make that happen. I would devote a two-hour time slot for her once a month for an outing to the mall. She would need to shower and put on clean clothes. We would have our other sessions either at her home or the office. And so it began. "To the mall therapy" sessions would start in two weeks.

Nadia was like an excited child that first trip to the mall. She had much to say about getting ready. Her daughter was equally excited about Nadia's mall excursion and they worked together the night before to choose her outfit.

"You are looking very nice today, Nadia," I commented as we met for our outing. She was in a lovely pants suit. Her hair was washed and styled and her make-up was just perfect.

"Thank you," she answered bashfully. She seemed to be looking forward to the outing, although she admitted to being anxious about being around people in a social setting.

"Well, let's just take it at your pace. If at any time you need to leave because it feels like too much, please let me know. Let's make this a good day, okay?"

She looked more relaxed as we headed to the car and off to the mall.

She and her daughter had mapped out which stores we should visit to start the outing. The plan was brilliant. We parked in the garage and started at Nordstrom's. We entered the store in the shoe section. She touched many of the shoes, talking about which ones would look nice on her daughter or son. We headed to the make-up counter as instructed by her daughter. After Nadia looked at a number of make-up brands, she boldly struck up a conversation with one of the saleswomen to ask if they had any free samples. Receiving a handful of cosmetics, she gleefully put them in the pretty bag they also supplied. Next, she went to the perfume area where she sprayed on a number of different scents with abandon. With her strong perfume presence, she also asked the salesperson at the perfume counter for free samples and was presented with a handful of samples she added to her pretty bag. With some amount of pride and a real and sincere smile, Nadia said, "These are for my Anya. She help me so much." She was so pleased that she would not be going home empty-handed.

We started our walk through the mall and stopped at Sharper Image (my idea) to try out the massage chairs. "Ahh" she purred as the rollers in the chair made their way up and down, massaging her neck, shoulders, back, and legs. "Your turn," she insisted as she enjoyed watching me luxuriate in my own chair massage. Amazed at the number of electronic gadgets for home, yard, car, personal care, etc., she commented as we were walking out, "We have to come here every month. I love that massage." Sharper Image was a hit!

We continued to visit the list of stores she and her daughter had mapped out. We found our way to the kitchen store and enjoyed having a number of free samples of dips and salsas with chips or pretzels. She loved that too. My favorite was going to the Lindt store and getting free samples of chocolate. She asked for a few extra and was able to take home a chocolate for her son and her daughter. "I love window-shopping!" she shared as we made our way back to the car.

I asked what she thought of our first outing as we drove back to her apartment. She had much to say about the experience. I was discovering a Nadia that none of us had met yet. She was animated and talkative, focused on something positive and enjoyable. She was even talking about plans for her future. What pleased her most was bringing home little treats for her children. We were both feeling that our first "to the mall therapy" session went quite well.

Very early on, one of the things I noticed with clients and therapy sessions which took place out of the box was how clients liked talking in the car. It always amazed me that clients who barely said a word in other sessions would have so much to say while riding in my car. I came to call this "parallel therapy." I called it that because we talked parallel to each other. It seems to me that clients who have self-esteem issues, high anxiety, thought disorders, and serious trauma don't like to look at you and don't like you to look at them. In a car, when I am driving, that issue is nonexistent. Both of us are looking forward to the road ahead. Paradoxically, that is when clients seem to be the most comfortable. All kinds of topics come up. Many of the conversations shared in my car were as therapeutic as any I have had in an office setting.

Nadia reminded me of how difficult it is when we find ourselves in a dark place emotionally. We plop ourselves down somewhere in that difficult emotional place feeling stuck and incompetent. Isolation becomes the norm and avoidance of others happens as negativity and self-loathing increase. While in that dark emotional place, we can't help but notice that others are out living their lives. We become afraid that we can't make it into the lighter places where everyone else seems to be doing just fine. My job with Nadia was to help her find a way out of her dark place and back into a life of relationships, connection, and happiness.

It reminded me of a time in my early adulthood when I was doing some backpacking. We were hiking across a snow field for a couple of miles. The only way to make our way through that field and towards the path we needed to follow was to look for red flags that were placed strategically through that snow field. Without those red flags we would have ended up walking around in circles, or veering off course because there was no clear indication of where to go.

My job with Nadia was to look for those proverbial emotional flags to help her back towards a better life path. Nadia was a woman of sincere and deep faith, as was I. I am sure that the God we believed in and trusted was guiding both of us so that Nadia could reclaim her belief that she was worthwhile. Where grace led me with Nadia was to first focus on the crush she had on her psychiatrist. That crush was all about wanting to connect with and please someone whom she valued. The conversation we had about her psychiatrist is what led to our "to the mall therapy." Starting with talking about her positive feelings for her psychiatrist provided that first emotional flag. Deciding to use our outings to work on finding more pathways to a healthier emotional life was another way to follow the emotional flags back toward a life she could appreciate.

We continued with our monthly "to the mall" sessions for four or five months. Her sister had started to provide her with a few dollars so Nadia could buy a little something or we could go up to the food court so she could take something home for their dinner that night. Our monthly shopping trips were a way to use something ordinary to find a value and a pathway to make the ordinary useful for her continued healing.

Our walks and talks were not the usual ones of friends and relatives who visit the mall. My focus was completely on her as I attended to her emotional and behavioral reactions as we made our way during those mall visits. Many of our conversations were about her thoughts, emotions, and reactions. As we walked and interacted, she was actively engaged in therapy. She was noticing in real time that she was able to recognize anxiety, negativity, and sadness and work through it then and there. I helped her to work on skills to strengthen her emotional and relational responses.

During the times that she would start to veer offtrack and get stuck emotionally, we could process it right in the moment. I would use a few questions such as, "What is the thought or memory that just came to your mind?" "Can you describe the emotion you are feeling right now?" "Is it time to feel better about yourself right now as you are experiencing something positive?" and she would use her thoughts and decision-making to choose a healthier response. I was helping her to notice those proverbial emotional flags on her own to get to a healthier life path.

She began to do better and her children were brought back into her care for several days a week. Eventually she became well enough to resume her full-time parenting role. As she had hoped, she started going to church. In time she even got involved with some church activities and got to know some of the other ladies there. In fact, there were some cooking opportunities at the church which were a big ego booster for her.

It was a blessing for her and her family that she made her way back to a life she could appreciate. She was beginning to be grateful for her decision to move to the United States. She came to the conclusion that this move and this difficult adventure became the most positive thing that had ever happened for her and for her children.

We noticed simultaneously that her counseling needs changed. The "to the mall therapy" sessions were no longer necessary. She was going on her own with her sister and her children. As her self-esteem improved, her anxiety and depression lessened. Talk therapy in a more traditional office setting was all she needed. We met every three weeks or so to check in, review progress, and discuss any continuing troubling thoughts and emotions.

In another few months, her individual counseling appointments had run their course. She had gotten what she needed from individual counseling. Towards the end of her time in therapy, she would share with me the antics and enjoyment of going to the mall with her family. She had reclaimed her joy in life and ability to connect with and be a part of the world again.

She reminded me about how important paths are. Getting us from one place to the other is what the path is all about. Our life path, or our life journey as some call it, is all about the lessons, the movement, the forward progress life is meant to provide for us. When life became too overwhelming for Nadia, she lost her way and got stuck on her path. How grateful I am that God was able to use me and some of my own life lessons and experiences so I could help Nadia to continue on her life path with more grace and happiness.

Nadia taught me about how important it is to be there for others. I was not the only one who was helping her to see the flags that helped to point her back to her life path. Her psychiatrist put out a few flags as he helped her find an adequate and helpful medication regimen. Likewise, her sister's devotion and love for her were a field full of flags pointing Nadia towards safety and purpose. As Nadia connected with other parishioners at her church, they also helped to plant some of those flags and confirm for Nadia that it is possible to find your way back even when it seems impossible. I was so happy to witness her moving ahead and finding her way to the path that was best for her.

CHAPTER 7

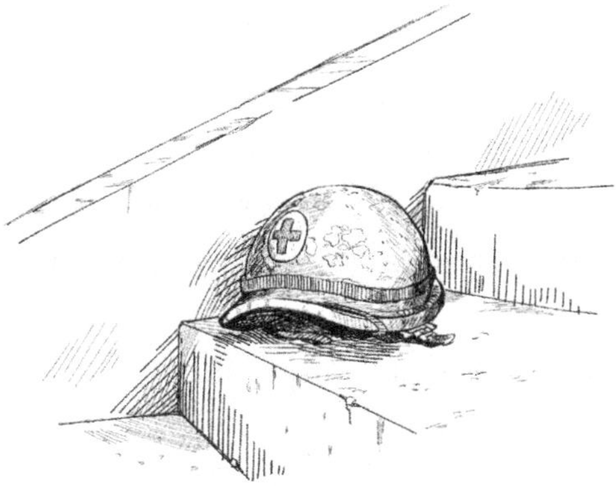

They Threw Me Out

I would try to get to the office early every morning. By early I mean that if work started at 8:00 a.m. I would try to be there by 7:58 a.m. It wasn't unusual that I would be the first or second person there. If I had to take someone to a doctor's appointment or we had court, I would be there even earlier. On this one particular morning I was actually at work around 7:45 a.m. I walked to the entrance of my workplace and there was one of the clients, Walt, sitting on the front step of our office building looking quite haggard.

We had just moved Walt into a new living situation about three weeks earlier. His assisted living home in our area had closed. With the help of our team, a newly built group home was found. Unfortunately, it was in a different catchment area. This meant that he would be living in a new town that was unfamiliar to him and working with a new treatment team who were unfamiliar with Walt. When we went to look at the new place, he was surprised at how nice it was. It even meant that he would be getting his own private room. That was a welcome and surprising bonus. The day of the move came. He moved in with much trepidation and excitement. We assured this good man that we would continue to meet with him and be available for a time to help with the transition. There was much anxiety about this change, but we did what we could to help him in his adjustment connecting with new people and new surroundings. We thought that the move had gone well as Walt expressed how nice it was for him to live in such a beautiful home. He had even found a coffee shop just a few blocks away where he could get an affordable cup of coffee once in a while. So, it was more than surprising to see Walt so early in the morning sitting on the front steps of my office building.

"Hi Walt. What are you doing here?" I asked.

"They threw me out of the group home," Walt responded quite despondently.

"Why? What happened?" I asked with much concern.

He was quite upset and confused as he explained that nothing had happened. The day before, he was minding his own business when staff approached him and told him, "You have to get out. You have to leave." So, he left. Since he didn't know any places in that area he decided to walk back to a place that was familiar. After walking about ten to fifteen miles, things started to look familiar. As the tale continued, he shared that he found his way to our area hospital. Finding the emergency room, he made himself as comfortable as possible and slept in a chair through the night. When morning came, he walked over to our office. That is when I happened upon him, sitting alone on the step looking quite disheveled and distraught.

I tried to offer some support to him regarding this challenging and confusing situation he was going through. We walked into the building and over to our office where I got him a cup of coffee and something to eat. I let him know that I was going to call the group home to get more information about what was going on. I would let him know what I found out. So, after he was comfortable in one of our counseling rooms with his coffee and snack, I called the group home.

"Hi, this is Celeste from MTT. When I came into work this morning, Walt was sitting on our front steps. He said that he had gotten thrown out of the group home. Did something happen?"

"Walt is there?" responded the group home staff. "We have been very worried about him. We had a fire drill yesterday at the residence and we didn't see him after that. We had no idea what had happened to him." They had alerted their area police station that he was missing but had not heard a thing.

"You had a fire drill?" I responded. I couldn't help but start laughing a bit.

We both figured out simultaneously that when Walt was asked to leave the residence for the fire drill, he could not make the connection that he was being asked to leave because of a fire drill, not because they did not want him there. I went to get Walt and invited him to join the conversation. The group home staff person and I explained that in his new home, unlike the previous place he had lived, they did some safety drills because they care about keeping all of the residents safe. Once he began to understand what had happened, he did relax quite a bit. With little encouragement from myself and the group home staff person, he agreed to go back to the group home. We made a plan that I was to take him back there later in the morning. Walt relaxed for a bit in our office, welcoming the attention of other staff who were so glad to see him, offering him more coffee and something to eat. It was good for him to get such a positive welcome.

Later that morning, Walt and I had a good ride back to his group home talking about what a big change he had just made. There was much to say about how every time things change it takes some adjusting to get used to new things.

During our ride Walt also revisited with me his regular stories of when he was in Vietnam working in the medical corps. His job was to rescue hurt soldiers. He would tell stories of running for miles with a wounded soldier on his back. He had many harrowing tales of how much he ran and how he would do it again in a heartbeat to save people. He would share these stories with so much pride in how he was strong enough in his younger years for that kind of work. "No one could run like I could run," he would say as he recounted the difficulties of running through the jungles of Vietnam. To him, it felt like that again last night walking all those miles. He just kept walking until something looked familiar and he was quite relieved when he made it to the emergency room at our local hospital. He was safe.

However, Walt was never actually in Vietnam. He never served in any war or in a medical corps. As a matter of fact, he had never had a competitive job. I met Walt in the early 2000s. He was in his fifties at the time. In his early twenties the delusions and hallucinations started. His behavior got bizarre and emotions were difficult to understand and control. He was experiencing psychosis, and was diagnosed with schizophrenia. Because of his mental illness, he was hospitalized at the State Institute for Mental Health. He spent quite a number of years there starting when he was a young man and well into his late thirties and early forties.

In those years there were not many options for treating mental illness and medications were crude. While the medications may have relieved some of the delusions and hallucinations, they would leave people feeling heavy and their minds groggy. It was almost impossible to manage the challenges and demands of adult life.

It seems that severe and persistent mental illnesses, thought disorders like schizophrenia and mood disorders like bipolar disorder, interrupt a person's life just when they are beginning to enter into adulthood. This is the time in everyone's development that they begin the process of becoming an independent person, ready to begin a life they create as their own. So many of the clients that I worked with earlier on in my career recounted how they were in college and got sick, or had started their first jobs or training program, or had just gotten married when the symptoms of their illness disrupted their early adult lives. They were initially hospitalized, sometimes for weeks and months. After discharge from the hospital, they would try to get back to their lives and would do okay for a little while, but the symptoms would return. Then another hospitalization ensued which resulted in loss of job, dropping out of college, and in some cases, marriages ended. All of the people I worked with were intelligent and remarkable human beings who had strengths and talents that enhanced their lives and the lives of others. The interruptions because of mental illness in some cases made it more difficult to reconnect with their strengths and talents.

Treatment for mental illness is so much better now than when Walt was a young man and first experienced the symptoms of his illness. That is the sadness of this disease, especially for the clients that I treated over the years who had spent time in state institutions when there were only inadequate treatments available. Over the years, as medications improved, and societal norms and approaches to treat mental illness expanded, it was no longer a life sentence of interruption and derailment. Treatments and deinstitutionalization afforded people the ability to live more independent lives. Many people benefitted from medication, community support, and opportunities to develop careers, enter into committed relationships, parent their children, and live their lives more on their own terms. Though, for a substantial number of individuals with chronic and persistent mental illness, life was challenging and maintaining employment or living independently were more aspirational than realizable.

I would like to think that if Walt's life had not been interrupted by his mental illness, he would have ended up in a career where he did help to save lives. He would have been good at that. He was the kind of man that always asked how you were doing and even though he couldn't always remember the answer, he always asked. He was kind and he had a good heart. He had a wonderful sense of humor and would come up with a good pun every now and again. With a thought disorder, that is evidence of sharp intelligence and quick wit. All those stories about his running through the jungles of

Vietnam saving lives may have, in some way, been a foreshadowing of who he wanted to be in his adult life. He wanted a career where he was working to help others, perhaps even to save lives. Wouldn't it have been wonderful if he could have pursued work that reflected the kindness and caring that were just part of who he was? I imagine that he would have walked many an extra mile to be there for others in his work and in his relationships to keep someone safe. The world needs more people like Walt.

The irony of this story is Walt was now in a place where people were working to help keep him safe. In this new residence all he had to do was walk a few steps to assure the staff he could be safe in case of a fire. Now that he knew he had a safe place to live with people who cared about him, I hope that he took walks when he wanted, relaxed when he needed to, and had people to joke with every now and again.

CHAPTER 8

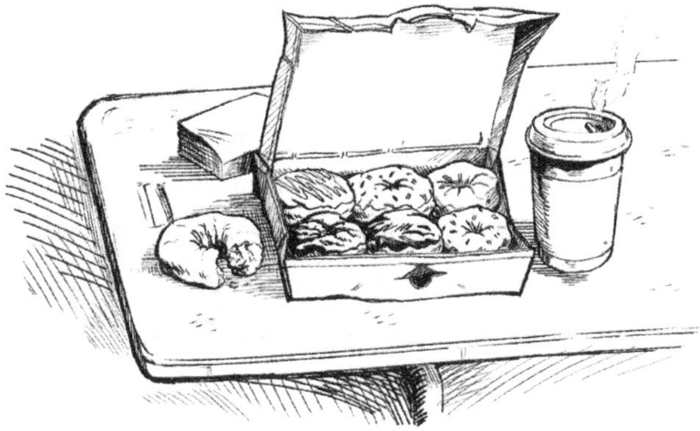

Have You Ever Had a Colonoscopy?

Early on in my career, a favorite supervisor asked and encouraged me to consider working with people with addiction and substance use problems in addition to their mental health issues. Despite some reluctance and fear on my part, I agreed. That meant taking some courses on substance use treatment and counseling for persons with addiction at our local college after work hours. I also participated in training to familiarize myself with resources for treating addiction. Attending peer led support groups was also something I did to learn about approaches that helped people with addiction issues.

So, I attended a number of Alcoholic Anonymous (AA) and Narcotic Anonymous (NA) meetings and Rational Recovery meetings, which are somewhat like AA but without the faith element. These meetings were very helpful in improving my understanding of what it is like to live with addiction and more importantly, to be in recovery. All of this improved my skill set and prepared me to better attend to clients with the dual diagnoses of mental illness and addiction. I sat for the exam and received a license in chemical dependency counseling to go along with my license in mental health counseling. I was stretched beyond imagination in taking on this challenge of working with people with addiction as well as trying to manage their mental health concerns. It necessitated much patience, compassion, and a sense of humor.

It is standard practice to use a group model in our treatment of those who struggle with their addictions. So, in one of the programs I worked in, we had two weekly group meetings our folks could attend. One in the early evening on a Tuesday, and the other on Thursday morning. The groups were well attended and many members were quite faithful to their group. There is something very healing about sharing your struggles with others who are going through the same things. Meetings were lively. There was much sharing including moments where tears were shed and group members who may have needed some extra support and attention were able to get what they needed for that week. We also laughed a lot as many of the members were able to share their life lessons in quite comical descriptions. We did not run our groups like AA or NA meetings but more like group therapy sessions. Staff would oversee the meeting and there was usually a topic presented that members could review together, addressing how the topic related to their own lives and struggles. It is a model with some proven success.

It was Thursday morning and my turn to lead the substance use group. For some reason, on this particular morning, I was running the meeting by myself. We tried to have two staff members co-facilitate when possible. This was especially helpful if something came up and a member may need individual attention. So, this Thursday morning, I would be handling whatever came up during the group on my own.

Staff would usually have some coffee and doughnuts or a pastry available for members when they arrived. It may have been an enticement, or a bribe to get clients to come, but it was much appreciated by attendees and it seemed to work. People showed up. So, the group assembled, got their coffees and pastry, and shared some idle chitchat about the weather or the latest sports scores. By this time most members were quite familiar with each other and always had something to say. On this particular morning, six middle-aged men in their forties, fifties, and sixties were present. For reasons unknown, none of our regular female members showed up that morning. It would be me and the guys in the group that day.

The custom of running group meetings ordinarily follows an agenda: check in, present topic, discuss topic, wrap up any challenging discussions, make plans for continued recovery, and review what is coming up in the next week. It seemed to work well and having an agenda that folks were familiar with could be helpful for discussions. So it was time for check-in and as usual, I brought the group around to focus on being together, thanked them for coming, and we started with our first check-in.

"So, Joe, how was your past week?"

"Well Celeste, it was a bit of a tough week. I went for my colonoscopy and it was just awful. Have you ever had a colonoscopy?" Joe went on for a bit of time about the exploits of the preparation, procedure, and aftermath of his colonoscopy. There was no way to stop his sharing and it got quite graphic.

So, when he finished, I responded: "Wow—that sounds really rough Joe—so glad that you survived to tell the tale."

Now onto the next member who did not miss a beat and began to share not only about his experience with colonoscopies, but also unnecessary information and details about other areas of gastric and intestinal distress. So followed the next member and the next until all six men were involved in very detailed and "gross" explanations, descriptions, and horror stories of bowel movements, intestinal and gastric distress, and the medical procedures to address these problems. It was just disgusting (and hilarious).

I did my best to corral the group back to the agenda with the response, "Well, it sounds like check-in seemed to land just on the topic of today—how to manage stress in recovery."

"You want to talk about stress," Tim (another group member) piped up. "I was so constipated once I could taste my shit! I went to the ER and I swear the doctor put a toilet snake up my ass—you wouldn't believe what came out—and the SMELL!!!"

Thus began another round with each male participant sharing their own horror stories regarding the texture and odor of their excrements. They also went into stories about various medical devices and procedures they had experienced that sounded quite torturous. They talked about medication disasters and home remedies that sounded just disgusting. They were on a roll and no matter how many attempts I made to redirect the conversation, I was not going to succeed. I had completely lost control of the group. The conversation had just gone south on the runaway shit train.

I couldn't believe it. What a complete disaster, so I surmised at the time. After the group was over, I made it back to the team room and was sitting at my desk a bit in shock, thinking to myself, What is it about guys and pooping??? It seems that whether a guy is eight or sixty-eight they just love toilet talk.

That was when another staff person asked, "So, how was the group?"

Not knowing what to say or how to respond, the only thing that came out of my mouth was, "It was a bit of a shitty group today."

The next morning during our meeting, we each shared our work from the previous day. This was our opportunity to discuss if there were any situations with clients or work that needed attention or support. As I shared about my substance use group and the colonoscopy debacle, I came to realize how actually funny the whole experience was. We all were laughing hysterically over the exploits of the "colonoscopy group." My fellow team members couldn't stop laughing and thoroughly enjoyed my recounting of the whole experience. As they shared their own silly comments and expounded upon the episode, it gave me a chance to rethink the success of that group.

That is the thing about group work: it can be quite tricky. Groups are about and for the participants of the group. So, while I may have felt and experienced being inadequate as the group leader for that day, maybe it wasn't about that at all. Maybe it was the group just being the group it needed to be for that day. If I may use a metaphor, the group leader is like the person who starts the engine and sets the course of the conversation more or less. Most of the time, everyone tends to follow the course of the conversation. Not so with the group that morning. It was like these guys were going on an emotional joyride and the conversation just went where it wanted to go.

The thing about it all, thinking about it years after, is these guys had a really good time with each other during that group. They all had much to say. They laughed and teased each other and were just enjoying being regular guys for a while. It is not unusual in groups that one or two people seem to say the most in the meetings—even when the group leader makes sure that each member gets a chance to share. But on that Thursday morning each member shared often and readily. They easily encouraged each other to share. Maybe, for this group, they were just regular guys talking with other regular guys. Maybe it was a moment to take a break from having to focus on the difficulties of addiction and the challenges of having to live with mental illness. Addiction and mental illness weren't part of the conversation on that Thursday morning. What came up was a time to share silly, personal stories, to make each other laugh and find a common experience they all shared.

After the coffee was all drunk and the last donut hole eaten, the substance use group wrapped up. One of our participants, Tim, said to me on the way out, "This was a good group today." And so said a couple more guys on their way out.

We laughed a lot during that shitty session. Those guys were hysterical and they were having such a good time outdoing each other about their pooping and farting! They left that session feeling quite satisfied. As the adage goes: laughter is the best medicine.

CHAPTER 9

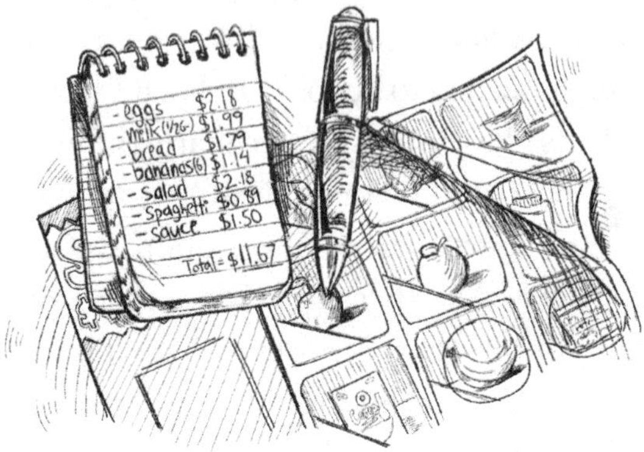

It Only Takes One Thing

I had the privilege to work on treatment teams for my entire career in community mental health. It is hard to imagine having done that work without the help, support, and input from colleagues over the years. There is so much we learned from each other. The feedback as well as the challenges from my colleagues helped in more ways than can be counted. They challenged me to be a better clinician, and a better person in the long run. This story illustrates how a simple comment from a caring and trusted colleague can affect just that little bit of an adjustment in attitude which then changes outcomes and improves relationships.

At the daily morning team meeting, we share our impressions of what happened with particular clients on the previous day and make plans for what we anticipate for the day to come with the clients we will be seeing. We also have a chance to ask questions and share important information about work, about ourselves, and about the resources, or lack thereof, in the community where we work. In the team meetings, we learn about new and interesting approaches to treatment and therapy. We share stories with each other about what we do, the essence of our work. Our work is unusual. It is work that not everyone is able to do. But for those of us who have worked in the field, the benefits are worth the challenges.

When you are the new person on the treatment team, you start by hearing from your colleagues about the clients with whom you will also be working. You get a sense of the culture of that particular team, work, and community. When I was working on support teams that provided home visits out in the community, my colleagues shared some pretty horrific tales of what a few clients were living through. As the new person, you would learn how difficult it is to work with some of the clients because their lives were so burdensome. These clients were impacted by the challenges of chronic and persistent mental illness, poverty, social isolation, addiction, and myriad daily trials. As the new staff member, you will probably work with the clients who are seemingly the most difficult and unpleasant. That is what happened when I was chosen to be the primary caseworker for Vinnie.

I first met Vinnie when accompanying one of my colleagues on a home visit. We were meeting at Vinnie's apartment. He was being evicted because of the horrendous condition of his apartment and because of his frequent outbursts. The outbursts were a result of the symptoms of his mental illness. His diagnosis of paranoid schizophrenia included realistic hallucinations and disturbing delusions. His most frequent delusion was that his neighbors were harassing him by sending him insulting messages through his refrigerator or the TV, or some other electronic device. He would shout and scream, pound on the ceiling with a broom handle or punch the apartment walls.

Vinnie was in a very foul mood on the day I met him. Screaming at us about how much he hated his apartment was our greeting that day. Raising his voice and speaking in vulgarities about his distaste for our work with him was his other theme. It was our fault that he had to move, he yelled, because we had done nothing to stop his neighbors from harassing him. About six feet tall, with thinning light brown hair and scraggly facial hair from not shaving for a few days, he spit out his complaints as he paced back and forth in the living room. His stomach fell over the dingy gray sweatpants he was wearing. The T-shirt on him may have been green at one time, though the original color had long been washed out, and his filthy sneakers showed a hole where the sock over his big toe was sticking out. There was a burning cigarette in an ashtray on the coffee table, and a second one he held in his right hand between his index and second finger. His fingertips were cracked and yellowed from the nicotine of his unfiltered, hand-rolled cigarettes and his fingernails were long, yellowed, and chipped.

Although my coworker introduced me, Vinnie completely ignored the introduction along with my presence as he regaled my coworker with his loud complaints. Vinnie's apartment was disgusting. It was filthy. It smelled of rotting food, smoked cigarettes, and dirty clothes. I could see the cockroaches in his kitchen walking over the unwashed dishes near the sink. There were mouse droppings in the living room and kitchen. A quick glance into the bathroom was evidence that it had not been cleaned in a long time. His coffee table was scattered with loose tobacco from rolling his own cigarettes. There was loose tobacco on the floor and couch as well. His furniture was ripped and damaged. There were holes in the walls where Vinnie had punched them during some of his outbursts.

My colleague's job that day was to inform him that all the furniture in this apartment could not go with him to his new place because it was too compromised. We were making arrangements to have the furniture removed and discarded. Plans had been made to get him some new furniture for his next apartment. That brought another outburst and more accusations. He was also informed that he had to take all his clothes and sneakers to the laundromat. They all had to be laundered and ready to go by the following afternoon.

We had large plastic bags with us and some money for him to get his clothes cleaned and bagged. With much complaining and swearing, he did agree to this.

When we returned the next day, his clothing was cleaned and bagged. He had done exactly what we had asked of him and he seemed a bit calmer. We moved him to his new apartment. It included furniture that was in very decent shape. Also, his new apartment was much closer to our office. We would be able to keep in better touch with him. I was reintroduced at that time, and better received as he grunted something like a "hello" my way.

You would think that I would have been completely grossed out and refused to ever go to his apartment or meet with him unless we were outside somewhere and I could spray him down with disinfectant or something. But it was never like that for me. Vinnie was not like that on purpose. He was ill. He had paranoid schizophrenia and was often bombarded and overwhelmed by a brain that was sending confusing, frightening messages. He heard insults and sounds and whispers that no one else could hear. If the refrigerator motor started, or the heat started, or there was static from the radio or TV, his brain would mistake it for something else. In his case, his brain told him that neighbors or people driving by were sending him messages from the CIA or the KGB that led him to believe he was not safe. Some of the people I worked with over the years lived in similar conditions. They did not qualify for home health aides because they did not have physical disabilities to warrant the service. There were not enough group homes or supported living situations to house people once the state psychiatric institutions were closed.

While many of our clients had family help and support, there was a group of clients who did not. While living independently was challenging for them there is no doubt they preferred this to living in a group home.

Vinnie was going to meet with me more regularly, now that I was going to be his primary caseworker and his therapist. He was very irritated about this. It was too much work to get to know anyone new, he said. He was so unpleasant at the beginning of our work together that I dreaded meeting with him every week. It was painful to have to bear his anger and unhappiness and it was very difficult to find a way to connect with him. Everything I said or asked upset him. My colleagues were supportive because their experience with him had been the same. No one wanted to have to work with Vinnie if they could get out of it.

It was my job to accompany him to do his grocery shopping. This would always be a longer than usual visit because it included a ride in the car, getting the shopping completed, and then a ride back to his apartment, plus some assistance getting the groceries put away. Oh dread!! He was waiting for me outside his apartment when I got there. He got in the car and said not a word on that car ride to the store. I followed him into the grocery store and asked if there was anything I could help him with. He pulled a shopping list out of his pocket.

The list was amazing. It was unbelievably well organized and put into categories that aligned exactly with how the store was laid out. Items on sale were marked on the list, and he had some prices indicated as well. This incredible list even had an estimate of how much he expected his groceries to cost at the end of the shopping trip. I was more than impressed. He asked me to get ketchup, including the brand and the size. When I had successfully gotten the correct product, I was given a few more items to pick up to help get the shopping done more quickly. On the way back to his apartment, I told him that I really liked the way he did his shopping. It was smart, organized, and well-thought-out. He said that he appreciated that. He also thanked me for helping him out. No one had done that for him before. So went our first grocery shopping trip.

The next day during our team meeting, I was happy to report that Vinnie was an incredible shopper. I described his shopping list and how we had a pretty decent conversation on our way back to his apartment. Joan, one of the nurses on the team responded, "It only takes one thing to make a good connection. Maybe you have found that one thing."

What a helpful, insightful, and positive comment! In fact, it was quite instrumental in growing the relationship between me and Vinnie. Who knew that grocery shopping would be such an easy opening to get to know a challenging man?

Vinnie was a person who definitely benefited from structure and consistency. He would anticipate the arrival of his food stamps and we would be sure to schedule a grocery shopping trip within a day or two of their arrival. Grocery shopping took place twice a month. He would always be prepared, so a helpful and pleasant routine was developed between the both of us. His job was to go through the aisles to get the groceries. Since he truly hated standing and waiting at the deli counter, I took on that task which was much appreciated. It is truly amazing that such a simple and benign activity meant so much to him.

Trust developed between us. On our rides back and forth from shopping and while we were putting groceries away, he would share with me so many things about his life. I learned that he had a girlfriend. Since he was such a difficult person, I was not expecting that. They met when they were both in the same group home after they had been discharged from Danvers State Hospital while many of the wards were being closed. Vinnie progressed enough to leave the group home and get his own apartment because he was able to take his medication properly and handle some adult responsibilities that she could not master. It was an on-again, off-again relationship that somehow worked for them. I actually got to know her quite well as she was often at Vinnie's apartment when I would arrive to meet with him. Vinnie was good to her, most of the time, as he would help with sharing cigarettes and going for walks and providing her a safe place to hang out when she needed to get away from the group home for a bit.

Vinnie shared much about his schizophrenia. I learned that it started during his adolescence and interrupted his schooling. He never completed high school. He continued to grieve the loss of his dreams and what might or could have been. We talked for hours about how difficult it was for him to move from the Midwest to New England with his father when he was a teen. He related how much he came to depend on him at that time. His father worked with horses on the horse racing circuit. They traveled up and down the East Coast during racing season. Vinnie shared a lot about how much he liked horses and animals. I came to understand quite happily that he wasn't so terrible after all. He was an interesting person!

Now, he was always a bit ornery. He hardly ever smiled and I am not sure that I ever heard him laugh. Even with his medication, he was haunted by persistent hallucinations and delusions. I worked with Vinnie for about five years and we still had to move him a couple times because of his complaints that the neighbors harassed him through his refrigerator. I never really figured that one out. He was almost never what you would call pleasant, but he became endearing. We became a good working team and it still amazes me that we grew to be so fond of each other.

Helping Vinnie to get a pet cat was one of the best things I could have ever done with him. He loved that little cat and did his best to take such good care of her. He was tender with her and he truly connected with her. He called her 200. He thought that was how much I paid for her when in fact, she cost nothing. That was her number at the pet sanctuary and was still attached to her collar when I brought her to him. I always got a kick out of the name he gave to her. It was very sweet to witness that side of this cranky man.

As trust developed, Vinnie even began to take my advice every now and again about all sorts of things. We worked on setting up a schedule for house cleaning and what products were better for cleaning his house. We brainstormed how to set up a schedule for taking meds and for recognizing when it was time to make an appointment with his doctor. We even worked on how to get along better with his girlfriend. They would have some pretty nasty disagreements which were quite stressful for him. She could be manipulative and cruel to him at times when he refused to give her cigarettes or money. He got better at setting boundaries and his girlfriend would meet with us to work on this as well.

It was not easy for Vinnie when I had some vacation time coming. The anxiety would build up and there would be some kind of an outburst. Even still, it gave us a chance to work on how to manage anxiety and recognize that he was perfectly capable of getting tasks completed with or without me.

The best thing that happened was that he began to connect better with all of the staff on the team. He was always a bit anxious and on edge, but he was able to control it better. He allowed himself to become more aware of his issues. He learned to talk about his anxiety and practice skills to lower it. Managing and decreasing his negative thinking also proved to be helpful for him. Most importantly, he had learned to do this with anyone on the treatment team. We had worked very hard on developing that skill. It made his life much better and more manageable. He was learning to be in relationships with people whom he didn't really know that well. He began to trust and believe that they were in his life for his benefit. My colleagues stopped complaining about him and started to look forward to spending time with him. That was quite amazing.

Vinnie and I did so many things together once the trust was formed. We worked on a plan to help to keep his apartment a bit more habitable. He was a terrible housekeeper and his apartments were often quite an atrocious mess. But he did work on this and his apartments did get a teeny bit more habitable.

He became more responsible about caring for his health and agreed to go to his doctor appointments. He had a number of serious health concerns that had been neglected for too long, including COPD, high cholesterol, high blood pressure, and obesity. While he tended to be consistent about taking medication, he was not consistent about going to appointments or would not follow up with recommendations from his medical providers. It took some time, but he did get better at being more responsible about his health needs.

Managing some enjoyable activities was also part of the treatment. There was this one particular park that he was especially fond of that included a bit of a drive to get there. We would try to go there at least a few times a year for some fresh air and a little picnic, bringing his girlfriend along with us to make it an even more pleasant outing. They loved music and would bring his boombox to belt out their favorite songs.

He eventually would even take some corrections from me if he was being especially vulgar or difficult. He would apologize and say, often, "I'm so sorry Celeste. I didn't mean to yell and swear at you." We would talk it over and try to figure out some ways for him to understand his anxiety and anger and to explore approaches to manage it better. He worked hard at this and made some progress.

Amazingly, all this happened because of that "one thing." Because my team member had given me that little bit of advice and encouragement, Vinnie and I were able to make a connection, and that "one thing" led to so many other connections. All those connections helped Vinnie to benefit from his participation in community mental health treatment. Vinnie had a chance to experience a better life for himself despite the daily challenges of living with mental illness.

We often make things more difficult than they need to be. Because I was trying to protect myself, I was missing those simple moments that challenged an unhelpful judgment. I got myself stuck in that awful "them and us" thinking. That "I'm okay, you're not okay" mentality. I spent too much time trying to protect myself from someone whom I didn't understand.

Honestly, I believe that God has other plans. God is so clever at helping us to get past the ridiculous barriers that we ourselves create. God put me with wonderful colleagues who were able to help me pay attention to how Vinnie did his grocery shopping! Sometimes it starts with just one ordinary thing that leads to a hundred other things that lead to a positive difference and a healthier relational experience.

Imagine that!

CHAPTER 10

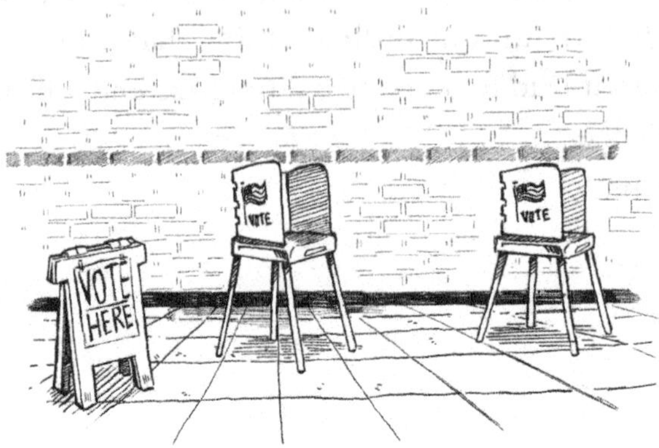

Today I Vote

It was the first Tuesday in November. I was working at a community mental health center doing counseling and community outreach. We had recently completed our morning team meeting.

Staff were busy getting ready for the appointments of the day. Some staff were catching up with each other about a client or scheduling issue. Most of us were at our desks. I was calling clients to confirm the day's appointments and checking my emails. While this was going on, Sam, one of my clients, came into the team room. What a sight as he entered looking quite dapper and dressed to the nines in his Sunday best. He wore shiny black shoes, pressed light brown suit pants and matching suit jacket, and a blazing white starched dress shirt with a lovely matching brown patterned tie. He topped it off with his best fedora hat.

"Wow Sam. Look at you!!! Are you getting married today or something?" says our team leader who was the first to notice Sam walk into the team room. The rest of us looked his way to observe his entry.

Sam responded with the biggest smile I had ever seen on his face as he proudly stated, "Today I vote!"

Sam was sixty-four years old. It was the first time in his life that he was casting a vote in an election. He was getting a chance to participate in the political process of his adopted country, a privilege never afforded to him in his native land. He was a recently minted US citizen. In the two previous years he took citizenship classes and worked very hard on improving his English.

Because of his hard work and determination, he passed the civics and English tests. His application for citizenship was approved in the past year. Over the summer he joined with other new citizens in a Rhode Island courthouse before a judge to take his Oath of Allegiance to the United States of America. Family and friends watched and witnessed as his citizenship became official. He was so very proud to become an American citizen.

There was so much appreciation for the freedom, indeed the responsibility, to participate in the political process. He did much to prepare himself for his first election. Reading as many newspapers and magazine articles in his native Portuguese as could be found and studying English newspapers to educate himself about the candidates and political issues were part of the preparation for his first election. He would be voting for a US president, a US senator, and a US representative. He was also able to vote for his local officials—mayor, city council members, and candidates for the Rhode Island House of Representatives and Rhode Island Senate. Excitement did not begin to explain the experience!

What a privilege to accompany Sam on voting day as I drove him to his polling station. We went into the school cafeteria where the voting would take place. As he checked in, he asked the polling official if I could go into the voting booth with him. Sam explained to them that since he had never voted before he needed someone to explain the ballot. The poll official did allow this as he accepted his ballot. We walked over to the voting booth. I showed him where the pen was to fill out the ballot and how to fill in the circles. I pointed out how the ballot was organized. He was amazingly attentive. I stepped out of the booth while he filled out his ballot thoughtfully, carefully, and indeed quite reverently. Upon completing the ballot, he picked it up and held it to his heart. That big wonderful smile returned to his face as we walked to the machine where he submitted his completed ballot. I was holding back tears as his smile broadened and he stood a bit taller. It was such a moving experience.

Let me tell you a little bit more about Sam. He was such a wonderful person, a gentle soul. He was a man of deep faith, strong emotion, and high intelligence. Born and raised off the coast of western Africa, he immigrated to the United States when he was in his fifties. He was sponsored by one of his siblings. His mother also immigrated to the US a few years before him.

As a young man in Cape Verde, Sam was conscripted to join the army. He received very little training and was put into the midst of a bloody and horrible civil conflict. He was severely traumatized from the experience. Very early into his involvement in the armed conflict he began to suffer from symptoms of PTSD, including uncontrollable anxiety, trouble sleeping, an overdeveloped startle response, and occasional delusions. At first, he was not allowed to leave military service because he had not suffered a physical injury. Miraculously, he did not have a severe medical injury but his psychological trauma was significant and penetrating. When he was released from military service, he was not able to manage daily life. He isolated, had nightmares, very little appetite, and minimal ability to participate in his daily life. He could not keep a job and was not able to support himself. His family did what they could to help but poverty and ignorance about mental health concerns left them ill-equipped to understand what was going on for Sam and get him the help he needed.

Sam was a very bright man who learned things easily. Loving to read and philosophize, even in the midst of his mental health symptoms he would read as much as he was able. Over time, with some distance from the trauma, he did begin to get better. Moving with family members to Europe, he spent time in Portugal and a short time in France. He spoke, read, and wrote in three or four languages. He learned a trade that afforded him the ability to make a decent living. With a good job and some stability, he was able to save some money and helped to send his mother to the US to join his sister. A few years later he had saved enough money so that he too could immigrate to the US.

Newly arrived in the US, Sam did the best he could. This was a difficult move. He could not speak English. Life was fast and complicated. In a matter of time the symptoms of his previous trauma began to emerge. He preferred isolation to company with others. In his lifetime he had never married or had children, which added to his isolation. He looked for work that was not taxing where he could work mostly alone. In a short time, the nightmares came back to the point where his sleep was regularly interrupted. The delusions and paranoia returned. His hallucinations and the outbursts he experienced scared his family members. He was hospitalized in a psychiatric hospital and started on medication. He stopped working and became even more isolated. His mental health symptoms increased, despite medication and more hospitalizations. After his last hospitalization, he was referred to our agency, to the mobile treatment team where I worked.

I was assigned to try some psychotherapy with him to address his ongoing PTSD symptoms. We hoped that this would help to provide some relief from his mental health symptoms. Now, Sam didn't speak much English when we started to work together. I didn't speak Portuguese. But we both spoke some Spanish and some French. And somehow between those two languages we were able to communicate as we began our counseling sessions. We spent hours in therapy sessions over a three-year period. As his mental health improved, his ability to understand and speak English also improved. Initially we met in a counseling office where he would talk and talk and cry and sob. At first, we focused on his mental health symptoms. He would tell me about his hallucinations and nightmares. Eventually, he was able to share about the horrors of his war experience. Once we were able to get to the real horrors and traumas, he could start to release the hurts and helplessness of that time. From there he was able to identify his real strengths and supports. At his suggestion, we started to get outside for some of our sessions, taking walks around the nearby track. The movement and the outdoors seemed to be very helpful for part of his healing. With the tears stopped and the fears released, he shared more and more about himself, his interests, and his hopes. He especially enjoyed sharing his philosophy about life on these very special and healing walks. These conversations helped him to connect with his more authentic self. He was getting better.

Sam never went back to competitive work, but he did much to help his growing extended family. He took up cooking for the family and looked after his aging mother. He was making a life for himself that he could manage. Life began to make sense for him.

Sam had enormous appreciation for the freedoms and responsibilities living in the United States afforded him. There was never an opportunity to vote, to express political opinions, or to participate in any political processes in his country of origin. He had been taught from a very young age to keep his thoughts to himself. "Don't rock the boat." "Do what you are told." "Don't speak up."

Getting used to freedom is actually quite challenging. Finding your voice takes some time. Sam had that in common with so many of the clients I worked with over the years who had been born and raised in other countries and cultures. Because of clients like Sam, including dozens of other international clients I worked with, my little world was expanded. It was as if the relationships that developed brought a certain kind of spark and interest to the work.

I had the privilege to work with a number of immigrants to the United States from Liberia, Uganda, Nigeria, and Cape Verde, as well as Portugal, Poland, and Russia. I worked with clients from Columbia,

Venezuela, and Haiti, and from the Central American countries of Guatemala, El Salvador, and Mexico. I experienced feeling appreciated from clients from the Dominican Republic and Puerto Rico as I tried to communicate in their native Spanish. It was truly a part of the work that was so very fascinating. It provided many opportunities to grow and stretch my cultural background. I loved it. I had to look for space inside of my brain and heart for curiosity, interest, and respect.

Adjusting to life in the United States was challenging for many of the clients born and raised in other countries or speaking a language other than English. My job as a therapist was to create relationships of mutual respect with clients with whom I had little in common. The work involved responding to whatever mental health challenge a client was experiencing. I wanted to affect some behavioral and emotional changes to help make their lives easier to manage. I am so grateful that my international clients were patient with me as I worked on getting my own cultural biases and expectations out of the way so that we could do the work that needed to be done. That seemed to be the lesson that I learned over and over again—pretty much every workday. I needed to get out of my own way.

What I learned early on in my work in mental health is that most clients will provide the clues and the pathway that will lead to a better emotional life. It was a matter of listening and finding my way to better questions. When I worked with clients like Sam, it necessitated more intentional listening. It also challenged me to find questions that would help me to connect with clients whose lives and backgrounds were a bit of a mystery to me. I wanted to know as much about Sam and the other international clients as I could. We talked about what they most appreciated about their cultures and upbringings. We talked about the family members they missed most and who most influenced them. Clients would share about how they celebrated holidays, what foods and practices they tried to continue and recreate here in the US. Clients loved it if I could speak a few words of their native tongue. Language connects people. It was important to understand that in each culture, language had its own particular powers of connection. As long as I stayed interested and curious, then the work of helping to improve someone's mental health concerns could happen.

Of course, what also happened is that I was changed. I grew in my appreciation of how brave and strong and determined these clients were. I cannot imagine how difficult it is to move thousands of miles away from what is familiar, learn another language, and adjust to whole new ways of being and surviving.

I believe that our diversity as a country is our biggest strength. Meeting clients from so many different cultures and backgrounds has been such an honor and a privilege. There are so many incredible memories of connecting with my international clients. I am sure that I benefited more than they did.

I grew up in Manville, a small mill village in Rhode Island that was probably of 80 percent French Canadian descent. In my youth, there were many families, including my own, where French was still spoken in the home and certainly around the village. My cultural experience is important and meaningful to me and I am certainly grateful for those experiences. Even though my initial exposure to cultural diversity was quite limited, there was a certain kindness and acceptance that seemed to be part of my growing years. I found myself fascinated and curious and wanted to know more about the backgrounds of my clients. And you know what? They wanted to know something about my background too. They were curious how I learned to speak some Spanish and French, and while the focus was on the clients, it meant something to them that I wanted to be able to connect with them in as many ways as we could find.

That is what is most important in the work I pursued. Curiosity, caring, and commitment to wanting to know another person are the most basic ingredients in mental health care. I learned that from the community that nurtured me in my youth. I also learned it from my international clients. They were in a difficult place emotionally. They were vulnerable and fragile in many ways.

I believe strongly that every human being is a treasured and loved child of God. It was imperative that I kept that in mind in this most important work, as relationships of help and healing are developed. What is most wonderful about that belief is that anytime one of God's children loves another of God's children a blessing happens for both of them. I think this simple but profound truth is probably what helped sustain me through decades of counseling work. In particular, with my international clients, it sparked meaningful connections with clients who felt disconnected and sometimes unwelcome and overwhelmed in this new country in which they found themselves. Part of the work with them involved helping them to feel welcome and valued. This sincere aspiration was integral in growing our counseling relationship.

The experience of working with Sam and especially having that incredible experience of taking him to vote for the first time in his life was transformative for me. How many people do you know get all dressed up like it is the most important day of their life to go vote? Until I had that experience with Sam, I had been taking the privilege and responsibility of voting for granted.

Now, whenever voting day comes around, I drive to my polling station, park my car, and as I am walking into the building, I try to stand a bit taller as I say to myself "Today I vote."

CHAPTER 11

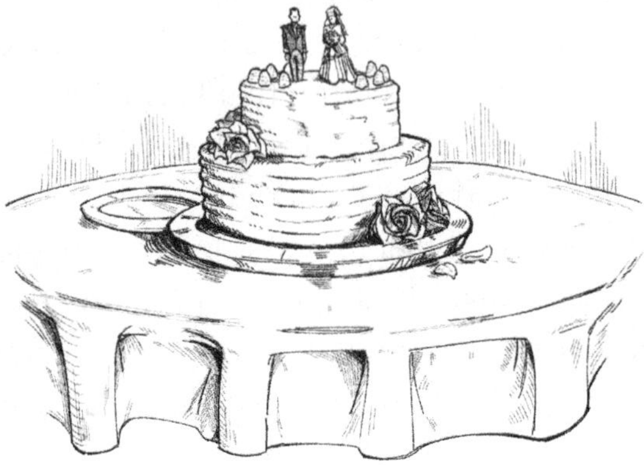

How Was Your Weekend?

There are a number of mundane and ordinary questions that we present to each other every day. "How are you?" "How are things going?" "What's up?" I suspect that the answers are also fairly ordinary and routine for most of us almost all of the time. "Fine." "Things are going." "Not much."

Every now and again, an answer from an ordinary question comes up that is quite unexpected.

It can take you a bit off guard. The following story presents just such a situation. After a very benign Monday morning meeting, I made my check-in call to my client Scott. Scott answered the phone with a lively "Hello."

I responded, "Hi Scott. How was your weekend?"

There was a momentary pause before I heard the response, "I think I got married this weekend."

My mind and imagination started to swirl with numerous scenarios as I took in that response. I thought to myself, What is he talking about? How could he not know if he got married or did not get married? Did he fly off to Las Vegas and hook up with a show girl? Did someone knock him out and he woke up with a ring on his finger? Was he drugged or duped into marriage?

At the time, I calmly responded, "What do you mean?"

Scott explained, "When I got home from work on Friday, Sue told me to hurry up, go take a shower, and put my suit on. She said that company would be here soon." Sue was Scott's roommate. The story continued that he went up to the bedroom where a suit was laid out on the bed. He took a shower and put on his suit. When he got back downstairs, guests had already started to arrive. A minister or some kind or a justice of the peace was there. He and his roommate, Sue, said some "I dos" and exchanged rings. Then they had a party. It did sound like he participated in a wedding ceremony where he appeared to have been the groom.

There were many questions I wanted to pose at the time, but decided it would be best to have this conversation in person. What I did ask him was if he wanted to be married and if he remembered any conversations with his roommate about plans to get married. The response was vague as he meandered through his confused thoughts, ending with saying he wasn't sure. However, he added, he was not unhappy about the situation. So, we made a plan to meet in person the next day to talk more about his new marital status.

We had been working with Scott for about two years. His primary diagnosis centered around being born with a developmental delay. Since childhood he had been part of special education services both in and out of school. His birth family was not always able to care for Scott and there were years when he was in the foster care system. In addition to his developmental delays, there were mental health concerns mostly associated with anger, hyperactivity, and some trauma history.

He was a delightful person who joined our program when he and his then-girlfriend (not his current wife) moved into our catchment area. Of African American descent, Scott was literally tall, dark, and handsome. He was thin and wiry and always seemed to be moving, which he seemed to use to his advantage. He smiled easily and endeared himself to people fairly easily. There were two things that Scott was especially fond of: work and women.

He always had great enthusiasm for work. His supervisors appreciated his energy and work ethic. He always had some kind of a job and was proud of his work accomplishments.

Scott also loved to be around women. Faithful and attentive to the women who became his partners, he worked hard to please them and look after them. On the other hand, Scott could be possessive and suspicious with his partners. When he became angry, he could become unreasonable and mean. No more than three months before this recent weekend marriage, arguments forced the end of his previous relationship. Police had been called and he packed his things and had to find another place to live. There were a number of concerns and worries regarding his current committed relationship. In particular, this marriage came about quite quickly.

What I did after the phone call was to meet with my supervisor and a few other staff who had a close connection to Scott. I shared with them what he told me about getting married over the weekend. All of us shared our worries and concerns. It is crucial to have colleagues with whom you can review what feels troublesome. Was Scott being taken advantage of? Was his new wife hoping to get her hands on his social security check and his work wages? How healthy was the relationship? Did she know what she was getting herself into? Scott could be difficult to be with, especially when he got angry. How do we respond to Scott with this new life reality without overreacting or underreacting? Of course, Scott has the right to marry and be with whomever he chooses. This was not what we were concerned about. Our concern was how to approach Scott without being judgmental or paternalistic.

Our peer specialist, Vivian, accompanied me the next day on that visit with Scott. Vivian was such a valuable team member. Her job was to share her own story, and to interact in very personal ways with clients to offer support and understanding. She also had a mental illness and had experiences that were very similar to those of many of our clients. As part of her recovery, Vivian had taken the time to participate in a peer specialist training and accreditation program sponsored by the State. This prepared her to work in the mental health field as part of a treatment team. I was always moved by the honesty, perspective, and compassion that she brought to the interactions and relationships that she formed with clients. I am so glad she was there that day. I was worried, Vivian was curious.

Scott was still on an emotional high when we met with him that Tuesday. He had much to say about the marriage ceremony and party from the weekend. He was practically jumping up and down in his seat. The emotion was contagious. We laughed with him and were touched by his obvious happiness. Vivian was the one who brought up the first concern. She asked if he wanted to be married. Again, his response was vague. I asked how he and his wife had made the decision to get married. Clearly it had been something that was planned ahead. He did admit that Sue had been talking about it almost from the time he had moved in with her. There was never a "no" or "let's wait" from Scott, so the wedding got planned and he happened to show up for it. I tried to bring up some of the concerns regarding finances and managing emotions.

The response was a sort of blank look. He emotionally retreated back into his confused self. But Vivian found a thread that made all the difference.

She brought up how grateful she was to have her father in her life. "We all need to feel like we belong to a family," she shared. She couldn't imagine how she would have gotten through all of the challenges of her life and living with mental illness if she didn't have her father there for her. The eye contact returned as Scott looked intently at Vivian as she shared about her gratitude for her relationship with her father.

Scott joined in the conversation. "I've known Sue since I was sixteen years old. She was a friend to me when I didn't have anyone. She took me in when Yvonne threw me out. She is the closest thing I have to a family. I want a family."

And there it was. "I want a family." That was what this was about. This was the reason for the happiness and giddiness he was feeling. Isn't that something that all of us yearn for? Isn't that something we all need? We have families that we are born into and families that we choose.

Scott had been without that relational reality for a long time. Our families are the biggest blessings in our lives, and provide many of the challenges as well. I know that I am a reflection of the family that helped to shape me. We can't become who we are without our families.

Of course, there are no perfect families. Nor are there perfect marriages. I have no doubt that there were many ups and downs in Scott's marriage. What was shared through Scott's giddiness and happiness was his belief that he had finally found his "forever family." That in itself is a tremendous blessing in anyone's life. It is especially helpful for people who are marginalized due to mental health issues, like what Scott had to live with.

Many of the clients that I worked with over the years were very much alone. There were many reasons for this solitary existence. Sometimes this was due to generations of social and mental health problems within the family. As such, some families just are not able to be the supportive presence that each of us need in our lives. Not all birth families are able to understand what is happening to the family member that has mental illness. Often, they will distance themselves from that person because they just don't know how to help.

In families that work at staying together, healing happens for everyone in that family. All families will experience challenges and learn many lessons. Anyone who is committed to their mentally ill family member will learn patience, negotiation, and advocacy skills. When a family member is experiencing the worst of their mental health symptoms, it is the parents, spouses, and siblings who bear the brunt of getting the medical interventions in place. They become experts in working with medical insurance companies and negotiating with medical professionals. They have a first-name relationship with social service agencies and mental health organizations. For the clients whose families stick with them, like in Vivian's case, they have a chance for a more sustained and healthy recovery. Families who get and provide support make a tremendous positive difference. As confusing and turned around as everyone's life becomes, families also create bonds and consistent support that no mental health or social service agency could ever provide in someone's life.

As our conversation came to its close, Vivian and I shared our best wishes and congratulations for Scott and his wife on that Tuesday. The three of us experienced a closer bond because of the opening of respect and understanding that Vivian created as we met and talked. What could have been a bit of a disaster, turned out to be an opening for hope and possibilities. Scott knew that if he needed someone to talk with about concerns regarding his marriage, he could trust that Vivian or I or anyone else on our treatment team would be there for him.

I am a sucker for happy endings. My family likes to tease me about how much I like the Hallmark Channel on television. "Those shows are unrealistic and too fluffy" they say. I respond that I look forward to that moment at the end of each movie where things work out. Hallmark shows are reliable and consistent in coming up with a resolution and happy ending to each show. And yes, they are very "fluffy."

In my work, there were many moments that were hard and sad. There were many times where words were inadequate, resources scarce, and resolutions not found. Many clients were very much alone. They persevered where they could. They made allowances and openings for the little bit of support and help that me and my colleagues offered. They all answered "How are you?" with the usual "Okay" or "Good" most of the time.

Scott reminded me to be open to anything that comes my way with his response, "I think I got married this weekend." More importantly, he helped me to appreciate that each of us brings something special to the work we do. Vivian was amazing in responding to Scott's fears and concerns. She found a way in and made a connection that was real and respectful. She made room for hope and the possibility that love can be healing and lasting.

We met a couple more times after that meeting as Scott had now moved out of our service area. As fortune would have it, he had also been hired to work in janitorial services at his local community mental health center which helped to connect him with the services he needed so close to where he now lived. When we had our last meeting, we wished each other well.

Sporting his new shiny wedding ring, he shared that he was as happy as he had ever been.

In my Hallmark, happily-ever-after mind, I hoped that Scott had found someone who was going to be there for him. I hoped and prayed that what Scott was feeling on that Tuesday lasted for many, many years.

CHAPTER 12

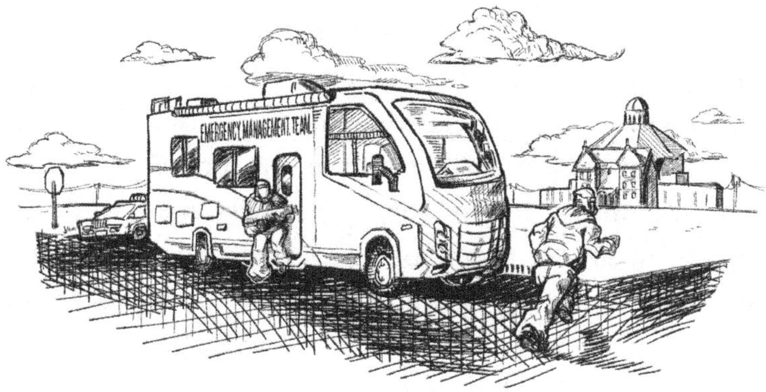

Trapped

One of the more unusual jobs in my tenure in community mental health work involved organizing and facilitating a federal grant that provided community-based recovery services for persons with addiction. It was a most fascinating job that required coordinating access to community services and supports for persons in need of recovery from addiction and mental health concerns all over the little state of Rhode Island. Our little state was fortunate enough to be awarded the grant along with a dozen other states to evaluate the effectiveness of services and approaches that provided comprehensive support to adults in recovery.

We worked very closely with the state department of mental health to identify the persons who would benefit most from the services we were promoting. One of those groups of people we connected with was composed of men and women in our state adult correctional facilities who were ready for discharge. All of them had been identified as having issues with addiction. Our services were put in place to help them have a more successful recovery and decrease recidivism.

I had access to seven adult correctional facilities. I was vetted, went through training, and then familiarized myself with how each of the facilities organized accepting visitors to their buildings. In particular, the training I participated in was for visitors who were offering programs to the inmates. Other persons in the training included clergy, educators, and other social service personnel. The training stressed how important protocol was and presented that there were no exceptions to the very strict rules afforded visitors to the facilities. You have to be there when you say you will. You have to dress sensibly and plainly—no fancy jewelry, high heels, expensive or flowy outfits. You cannot bring anything into the facility except what is allowed—no purse, no cell phone, no jewelry, no identifying information like where I lived, or pictures of family members. In my case I could bring my stack of assessment papers that needed to be completed and signed by the inmate with whom I was working that day. I could also bring one pen. No paper clips, staples, or file folders were allowed. Just me, my papers, and one pen. I would also have to show the correctional officer on my way out of the facility that the one pen and stack of papers were leaving with me. I literally came face-to-face with what happens when rules are not followed; one of the inmates I met early on in my work there had been recently stabbed in the eye with a pencil by a rival gang member. They lost sight in that eye. I followed the rules.

There were set times when we were allowed to enter the facilities. We had access in the mornings from 9:00 a.m. until 10:30 a.m. and in the afternoons from 1:00 p.m. until 2:30 p.m. In that one and a half hours you had to get to the room provided for you, wait for the correctional officer (CO) to bring the inmate to the room, and then rush through an assessment that was designed to take over an hour. In addition, I would then hurry the inmate through the signature process so I could be back at the service desk by 10:30 a.m. or 2:30

p.m. when all visitors had to leave. It was so nerve-wracking. Besides all that, you had to go through any number of locked doors to get to where you needed to go. I was as locked in to that facility as anyone else, except for the inmates.

I would arrive around fifteen to twenty minutes before we were allowed into our meeting space with the inmate with whom I was meeting. I would have to wait in line to meet with the CO in charge of entries for that day. I would be given a key to a locker for my personal items, or I would hand over my coat, purse, keys, etc. to be locked up behind the desk. The CO would also look through anything that I was bringing into the facility and confiscate any non-allowable items.

One of my more memorable experiences at the adult correctional institute happened on a very beautiful October morning. While the buildings themselves were imposing and scary looking, the grounds of the complex were quite lovely. There were well manicured lawns all over the campus and the trees that were on the grounds were in their full autumn glory on that exquisite morning. Red, auburn, yellow, and green leaves swayed when gentle breezes moved them and put on quite a show.

The building I was visiting that day was one of the women's facilities. I parked my car in the parking lot and approached a large brick structure with small windows and wrought iron bars in front of each one. There was a high chain-link fence with razor wire along the top that started on either side of the building and went around and to the back. In the back of the facility surrounded by the same chain-link fence was a small courtyard that was used by inmates at designated hours.

I entered the building and made my way to the front desk. There were very few visitors that particular morning so I was at the desk quickly. By this time, I knew most of the COs at the entry desk. I had gotten used to the routine of the ins and outs of the buildings. As she took my coat, purse, and car keys, the CO informed me that a training drill was scheduled for this particular morning at 10:30 a.m. She suggested that I do everything I could to be out of the building no later than 10:28 a.m. or I would be locked into the facility for as long as it took to complete the drill.

Oh brother, I complained to myself as I verbally agreed to the request. There was barely enough time to get through everything as it was and believe it or not, two minutes was quite valuable in helping to complete the assessment process. The inmate and I rushed through the assessments and with determination we finished in time for me to get back to the desk by 10:28 a.m. The CO had my things ready for me with a "You'd better hurry," as I rushed out of the building. My foot hit the outside step of the building just as the sirens for the drill went off. I practically jumped out of my shoes. The siren was SO loud. Thankfully I made it out just in time.

I walked across the circular driveway to get to the parking lot. In a matter of seconds—and before I reached my car—vehicles started to arrive. The drill had started. Sirens were blaring and lights were flashing as three enormous motor home-looking vehicles raced down the road and into the circular driveway. The vehicles' signage indicated they were from the state emergency management agency. The state headquarters for the emergency management team was just across the street from the adult correctional institute. Hence the quickness of their entry. A number of fire apparatuses, ambulances, and police cars, also with sirens blaring and lights flashing, rushed into the circular driveway as well.

Getting into my car, I noticed people began to emerge from the large motor homes as more vehicles arrived. Most of the people who emerged from the emergency management vehicles were dressed in orange dayglo jumpsuits. There were so many of them! They had their hoods up and were putting on goggles and strapping oxygen tanks on their backs. They even had on matching dayglo slippers for their feet. A few people were putting up a white canopy and a couple of long tables were set up underneath. Some monitors and other electronic equipment were set up on the tables and orders were given as the dayglo creatures ran towards and into the facility.

"What the hell??" I said out loud as this incredible procession of emergency vehicles and emergency personnel took over this spot and blocked me from exiting. Before I knew it, the parking lot was completely surrounded and all exits were blocked. In a matter of seconds, I was trapped!! There was no way out of the parking lot. I sat in my car for a while witnessing this most unusual occurrence. It looked as if a real and horrible emergency were taking place, as if toxic gases or radiation were just released into the air and in a matter of seconds, we would all be dead! Except for the dayglo creatures who were dressed for such an awful event; the rest of us would all be goners.

This was a most unfortunate situation, I mused. Deciding to let someone know what was going on, I reached out to my admin assistant on my cell phone. It entailed a rather detailed and lengthy explanation as I described the dayglo creatures, the flush of activity, and all of the apparatuses blocking my exit.

"What do you want on your tombstone?" she joked with me as we contemplated my untimely demise from the imagined odorless toxic gas that was being released right where I was parked.

"Ha, ha, ha," I responded back. "I am not sure how long this drill will take, but I hope it will be over quickly." The cell phone conversation ended and in my uninformed mind, I thought the drill would be over in a short amount of time. I had my laptop with me and my recently completed assessment so I started to put the information into my laptop as the drill continued. Thirty minutes went by and all of the vehicles were still parked in their original spots and still blocking the parking lot.

Exiting my car, I looked to see if there was someone whom I could approach about moving a vehicle or two so I could get out of the parking lot. Spotting a policeman who was just standing around seemingly doing nothing, I approached him and told him of my situation, asking if it would be possible to move a vehicle so I could get out of the parking lot and on my way. He said he would see what he could do. Glancing around, I found a grassy, shady spot to sit and view the goings-on. I settled down and made myself comfortable as I continued to monitor this situation. Even though I had my laptop, there was no access to the internet so getting things done was limited.

Another half hour went by and still no movement of vehicles. I approached the same policeman to inquire if he had an idea of how much longer I would need to wait. He had, in fact, not asked about moving any vehicles but responded that he would go to talk with someone at the command center presently. He walked toward the long tables where the command center was located and looked back to see if I was watching. I was.

Now, it wasn't as if everyone was in dayglo outfits and responding to the imagined emergency. There were quite a few people just standing around in small groups in their everyday uniforms, talking and doing whatever people do during an emergency drill. My admin assistant called a few times to check if I was still breathing as she found the situation endlessly amusing.

Another half hour went by and again I approached the unhelpful police officer. This time all I said was, "Well?"

"They will be moving vehicles very shortly," he responded.

I went back to my spot, and although I was quite annoyed, it really was a beautiful day and having a moment to sit and just be was not really all that bad. With no ability to get work done there was time to just sit and observe and think. I had a chance to give an honest appraisal as to what it was like for people who actually are trapped. Being incarcerated is all about being trapped. They were trapped in their buildings, in their cells and in the daily mundane routine incarceration entails. Those inmates were trapped by the poor decisions and behaviors that led to their incarceration. Many of them were trapped by the circumstances of addiction that led them to compromise who they were because of their addictions.

Some of them were trapped because of the challenges of poverty that limited opportunities and pathways to a more successful life. Sometimes choices were made that led to connections with gangs and illegal activities as a way to make some money. They hoped that with some money they could find a way out of their situations. They dreamed of affording a better place to live, a better life for themselves and their children. Being associated with gangs became another entrapment for unsuspecting new members. Unfortunately, they became entangled in gang life and beholden to the gang and gang expectations.

The men and women I met were stuck and trapped by the circumstances of life where they pursued a path that was doomed. Some people decided that they were smart enough to get away with cheating and stealing, until they actually got caught. Many of them would blame the people who caught them trying to justify their behavior by stating they didn't hurt anyone. The trap in that scenario is the lies we start to tell ourselves and then believe. Accepting responsibility for hurtful and selfish decisions takes a good deal of honesty and courage. It can start someone on a better and more meaningful path, especially when chances for help are presented.

Meeting and interacting with inmates was having an impact on me. Many conversations about hopes for a better life were shared as opportunities were identified to realize some of those hopes. That is what I offered them when we met for those assessments. Our grant offered housing and employment assistance for up to eighteen months for those who needed that help. There was also money available for substance use counseling, mental health counseling, and medical care. Much emphasis was also put into individual peer support so that all who took advantage of the program could benefit from mentorship for a more sustained and successful recovery. The grant was a chance to assess how effective providing comprehensive support for people struggling with crippling addiction could be.

I thought about the woman I had met that morning. She had embezzled money from her workplace to support her cocaine habit. She had been incarcerated for quite some time because of her crime. Through much hard work she maintained her sobriety and grew in her recovery throughout the incarceration. Alcoholics Anonymous and Narcotics Anonymous meetings were what made the difference for her and she faithfully attended and participated in meetings at the facility. Following the program was helpful. Meaningful connections were made with program members from the outside who came to run the inside meetings. In fact, they encouraged her to ask for help from my program. It was impressive how well prepared she was for our assessment that morning. Her story was inspiring as she shared about her current sobriety and desire to continue her progress. We can't underestimate how important it is to ask for and accept help.

She was prepared for both at our meeting.

In my silly little situation that morning, I also had to ask for help. Asking for help is not easy. Being stuck is not easy either. It bothered me that what I asked of the policeman was not at all a reflection of something that was wrong with me or my life or my choices. My request to move a car or two cost him nothing and did nothing to disturb his work, or his day. I made a simple, reasonable request and I had to ask more than once. Not only that, he was rude and treated me like I was an annoyance.

In my work over the years, I witnessed how much strength and persistence it took for my clients to ask for the help they needed just to survive. Applying for SNAP benefits, housing assistance, utility help, or managing social security benefits is quite complicated. The number of documents you need to gather and present is significant. Managing to get an appointment is almost a full-time job. It starts with making a phone call which literally takes hours and occasionally several days to get through to someone. Clients often wait for an hour or more in the waiting room to see their worker, even when they have a set appointment date and time. The appointments are long and the paperwork is substantial. The qualifications are numerous and there are no exceptions. Getting any kind of government help is hard, time-consuming, and humiliating. That being said, the government workers we met were mostly kind and respectful to the clients I accompanied for these appointments. They appreciated that there are people going through hard times and they were trying to help. These workers were also limited by the demands of their work. Over the years the requirements to apply for assistance have become unbelievably cumbersome. I suspect that this is mostly because of the false narratives of so much "fraud and abuse." The clients I accompanied to these appointments had chronic illnesses that impacted their ability to work competitively. They were not able to support themselves through work and the only way for them to survive was to seek out government assistance.

It hurts my heart when I hear people making harsh judgmental comments about people who use SNAP benefits or who are on housing assistance or getting SSI benefits. It just galls me when I hear someone making the comment that all people on SNAP benefits buy steak and lobster and are taking advantage of hardworking Americans. I literally went into the homes of dozens of people on SNAP or housing assistance. The people I visited and spent time with had very simple lives and they learned to live on very little. I never witnessed anyone feasting on expensive meals with SNAP benefits.

My clients did the best they could with what they had. Illness and poverty are double whammies. No one I worked with imagined their lives would be what they had become. No one wanted to be ill and they certainly did not want the poverty and challenges that chronic illness or disabilities bring. No one deserves wealth any more than any of the clients I worked with deserved illness or poverty. That is one of the hard truths of life. There is a capriciousness in why some people have the blessings of good health, access to opportunities, good paying jobs, and generational wealth. Others start out behind from the start being born into poverty, a lack of opportunities, and dead ends as it seems our society systemically leaves behind segments of our population. We would like to think that life is fair and that all of us get a fair shot at opportunity and wealth.

That just is not always the case. That silly experience of being trapped on the grounds of the adult correctional institute brought me face-to-face with this lesson of advantage and disadvantage.

Our society is often at odds about services for those who are disadvantaged. There is so much disinformation about entitlements and help for those who are the most disadvantaged. There is the myth of welfare queens and how there is uncontrolled fraud and abuse. That just is not the truth. The amount of cruel and uninformed statements about people who get government assistance is truly undeserved. I am not saying that there is absolutely no abuse of the system. I am just recounting my experience of accompanying so many people through hard and difficult lives who were not abusing the system. They truly needed and benefitted from the help. It seems to be human nature that we complain about the inefficiency of the federal, state, and local governments. We forget that we are all connected and brought together because we live in a certain country, state, and municipality. We all have a part in how the government responds to the needs of the people in our country, in our states, and in our local towns and cities. When a society and government choose to help those who need help, that is a good thing. Everyone benefits when we look out for each other.

It is not an accident that most people who have done service with the marginalized and disadvantaged come to appreciate that neighbors helping neighbors is what our system of entitlements is really all about. That it has become institutionalized within our governmental systems is what needed to happen. Sometimes those neighborly responses need to be national and then filter down to each state to support those who through no fault of their own are ill, develop the awful condition of addiction, or try to manage life with disabilities. The little that is provided goes a long way. Acknowledging that we can do more and finding ways for that to happen are much appreciated by those who benefit from the help offered.

That grant program I worked in for four years was helpful and successful. Our follow-up work indicated that a majority of those who participated maintained recovery and sobriety for many months. Work was found and maintained. Having a safe and sober place to live with consistent peer support was undoubtedly a key ingredient in their better lives. What we were able to provide was making a positive difference. It was gratifying for all of us who worked with the grant.

I do know from my experience that when information regarding the needs of our disadvantaged neighbors is accurate and reflects respect and compassion, we know how to respond accordingly. We help. In this blessed, generous country of ours, let's keep finding ways to be there for each other. Let's be more honest about the difficult changes we need to make so that all people cannot only survive but thrive. We think that it is expensive, but it is not nearly as expensive as leaving people behind in hurt and want. We aren't nearly there yet, but my hope is that we keep on working to get closer to that goal. As we know, being trapped is a ridiculous and awful experience. Maybe there are ways that all of us can help to recognize and reduce the unnecessary traps that too many of us get caught in.

CHAPTER 13

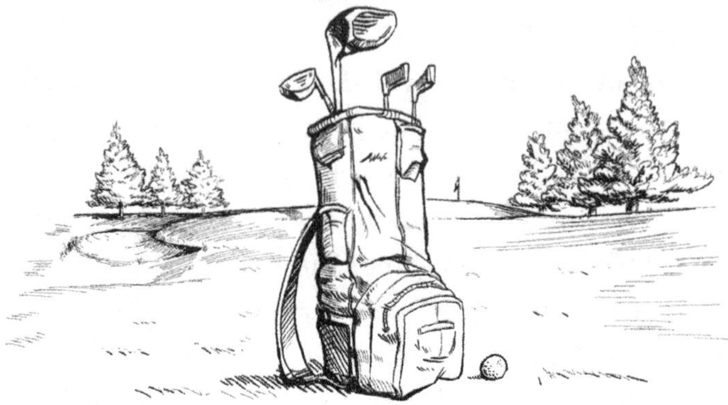

It's All About the Plan

I worked in community mental health for about thirty-eight years altogether doing a number of diverse jobs over that time. In the last ten years of service one of my duties was to work with adults who had been charged with driving under the influence of alcohol or drugs, a DUI. They were court-ordered to attend substance use counseling to meet the court's requirements and, in most cases, in order to reinstate their driver's license. It is the one time in my career when I met people with a wide range of backgrounds. Almost none of them had a chronic mental illness.

Of course, I do not in any way condone anyone who gets behind the wheel intoxicated or impaired by alcohol or drug use. At this point in time, there are many options for anyone who drinks more than what is safe to operate a vehicle. Drinking and driving does not have to happen. I have been inspired by groups like MADD (Mothers Against Drunk Driving) and SADD (Students Against Drunk Driving) and other community advocacy groups who work at raising awareness. What they do does make a positive difference.

It amazed me that counseling these clients became a rather interesting part of my work. For many of those court-ordered for treatment, this was their first counseling experience. It was a surprise for almost all of them that they actually didn't hate it. As a therapist, it is quite gratifying when a client appreciates the work done and relationships developed during our counseling sessions. In fact, one of those DUI clients with whom I worked made a profound impression on me.

One day a middle-aged man presented at my office for substance use counseling. Physically an unimposing man, with a ball cap on his head to hide his receding hairline, he presented at his first appointment as just another average Joe. However, his pleasant, open personality and ability to engage with focused eyesight and an easy smile helped to form a valuable connection. I learned that he was a professional businessman who was very well-respected in his field of work. With a responsible and well-paying executive job, he developed enough prestige and privilege in his career that he had time to golf a couple times a week at his country club. After his golf outings, he and his friends would spend time in the clubhouse to have a few drinks. It was after such an outing that he was stopped by police and found to be driving under the influence of alcohol. He was charged with a DUI. In order to meet his court requirements, he would be participating in counseling services for the first time in his life.

I'll call him Pete. From our first meeting it was clear that Pete definitely thought he had better things to do with his time than come to counseling. Quite frankly, the majority of the clients I met with for DUI substance use counseling came with a similar attitude. I was not surprised by this. At their first meeting many of them claimed they had been targeted by the police and had done nothing wrong or dangerous. For almost all of the people I worked with over those ten years, these thoughts usually started to change as the appointments progressed.

With Pete it was different right from the beginning. Although he was not that keen on having to attend counseling sessions, he was aware that he had done something irresponsible and unsafe. He should not have driven a car while intoxicated and he did accept the consequences of that decision. The requirement to reinstate his license necessitated he attend ten counseling sessions. There were topics for each of our appointments that addressed concerns related to substance use and intoxication. The meetings immediately became a sharing back and forth that made the experience very interesting for me.

From the second session on, Pete became a bit intrigued with the topics and the discussion they would raise. We addressed the risks of intoxication, the science and biology of intoxication and addiction, genetics and family patterns, how change happens, the purpose of emotions, and the challenges of intoxication and decision-making. Curious and intelligent, Pete would ask questions eagerly, welcome debate, and share insights as they were developing in his mind.

Relating the topic to his work and life happened readily, which enhanced the counseling experience. He always started our discussions acknowledging that he had things to learn and made it a point to relate our topics to his everyday life. He taught me about management and sales, motivating people, and the power of communication in the business world. His understanding of basic human psychology was well formed and thought out. It was fascinating for both of us because we learned from each other's different experiences and life lessons.

Something in particular happened when we were working on the topic of how change happens. This topic has to do with the reality of change in all of our lives. Change happens when life introduces either positive or negative and planned or unplanned life experiences. For example, we graduate from high school or have a child, or in Pete's case, get a DUI, which in each scenario will bring about a life change. He began to notice that he saw his DUI experience as a chance to learn the importance of recognizing and taking responsibility for mistakes. We were talking about the importance of "the plan" when change is coming or has happened. He said rather benignly, "My wife tells me all the time that 'It's all about the plan.'" I responded that he was very fortunate to have such a wise wife. "Yes, I am," he said. And I believe he meant it.

This tidbit of knowledge followed us through the rest of his counseling sessions. When we explored the purpose of emotions, discussing guilt, embarrassment, and regret, he provided a very honest look at how he had tried to avoid these emotions. It is painful to look at our faults and mistakes. Yet again, Pete made the connections between what we had been discussing and relating our discussions to his own life. He wanted to know about his mistakes, because, with that knowledge, he could put together a better plan. He understood that it is not just about acknowledging weaknesses. It is about understanding them, evaluating them and coming up with a better plan to avoid making the same mistakes. The humiliation of the DUI reminded him that he did something stupid, irresponsible, and dangerous. If he didn't change something, it would happen again. Fortunately, he had the input of his very wise wife to remind him that if there is a kink in the plan, you change the plan. You update it. You revise it. You come up with a better plan.

What this experience brought to Pete's mind in technicolor was the importance of his values: who and what matters to him. It is only because of what matters to us and what we value that we can feel and experience guilt and regret. Without the ability to know what is important to us, we miss out on real and sustaining growth. A parallel truth is that what matters to us and what we are connected to are what bring real joy and happiness into our lives. That is what the emotion of happiness reminds us of. What brings real and lasting happiness are the people, the pets, the natural world, and our interests, values, and beliefs; things we are connected to. What sustains our happiness are the principles and values by which we live. When we explored the emotion of gladness, Pete was able to relate easily to his connections and values. He recalled the emotion he felt when his children were little and jumped into his arms, exclaiming excitedly, "Daddy's home!!" That experience is difficult to put into words. However, the tears welling up in his eyes left no doubt that he had experienced real and tender love in his life.

He was fully committed to growing that love as his life and relationships matured. He was recognizing what mature love looked like now that his children had entered young adulthood. He and his wife were entering into a new phase in their marriage as they were about to become empty nesters. For him, mature love reflected the importance of the strong ties that he had developed carefully and intentionally over the years.

The experience of getting a DUI reminded him that it does matter what you do with your time and with your opportunities. Careless mistakes can easily derail anyone from a path that had been taken for granted. He was taking some time, through this experience, to first of all be more mindful of what and who was important to him. Understanding the importance of taking responsibility had been a central value throughout his life. Decisions and actions have consequences. Pete wanted to have more positive than negative consequences in his life going forward, if he could help that in any way.

When we had come to the end of our counseling sessions, we had a meaningful parting as we thanked each other for what we had learned from one another. Pete was relieved to have this experience behind him. In a short time, his license would be reinstated. Before he knew it, he would have his life back as before. Although maybe not quite like before. When we have these growth opportunities, there is always a bit of us that stays more alert—or enlightened, if you will.

It is amazing to me how much Pete's openness to this counseling experience affected me as well as I reflected on the power of change and decision-making in my own life. He reminded me of how to put the Serenity Prayer into action. I always had a cross-stitch of the Serenity Prayer hanging in my office:

God grant me the Serenity to accept the things I cannot change,
The Courage to change the things I can,
And the Wisdom to know the difference.

The sentiments in this short prayer are quite profound. For so many people, it is a reminder to ask for the help of serenity, courage, and wisdom, especially when troublesome life experiences derail our life a bit.

If I had not effected a change in my own life, I would have never met Pete. Ten years earlier, I had gone through a divorce that I neither wanted nor anticipated. At the time I was left adrift in just about every area of my life: emotionally, financially, and relationally. Because of that unexpected change I had taken on a leadership position at the community mental health center where I was working to increase my income. For two years I worked in a position that I neither wanted nor sought out, becoming more unhappy and emotionally unhealthy as the months went by. Making a change and effecting a better plan were becoming a necessity.

The Serenity Prayer helped to wake me up and lead me to that better plan. I prayed daily for the serenity to accept what had happened that I could not change. I was divorced. I now needed to create a life for myself that would make sense and leave me safe and happy. Not knowing what the change would be, I prayed for courage and wisdom to recognize how to make and effect this change.

One morning, during that trying time, while watching the news as I got ready for work, a feature on the broadcast announced a help wanted ad for a master's level clinician to work at a mental health center. That center happened to be just seven miles from where I lived. A résumé and letter of interest were sent out to the agency. Within a short time, they contacted me and asked to schedule an interview. On my way to that interview a most unusual thing happened. Just after I traveled underneath the overpass for Route 99, an eagle flew right over my car hood directly in front of my windshield. The eagle was huge and the wingspan was impressive. It was startling and beautiful. I pulled over for a minute to take that in. It felt so much like a sign, a confirmation from God: "I will raise you up on eagle's wings, you shall run and not be weary, you shall walk and not faint." (Isaiah 40:31). A surety developed inside of me for that day knowing that courage would be there when I needed it and I would know what to do.

The interview went very well. Within a month I was an employee at Family Resources, which became the best work experience I ever had. That would be the last résumé I would ever send. Here the remaining days of my work life would play out within this agency, which in a few years became the Community Care Alliance. That was the best plan I had ever made and enacted.

In essence, Pete and I were actually working on how this prayer can be more a part of our lives. There is no doubt that life will present us with numerous opportunities to put the Serenity Prayer into practice. We make mistakes, we fall short of using the talents and gifts we were given to make a positive difference in our relationships and in our lives. For me, I take things for granted. I just don't bother with being there for others, or for myself sometimes. I opt out of the lessons I actually need to learn that challenge me to be wiser and more courageous.

And then, I meet someone like Pete who helps to remind me of the importance of the plan. He moved me to remember and to be grateful when we have chances to put our plans into action. On my bulletin board I had created my own version of the Serenity Prayer, with a little change in the wording. This is my take on how a small change can make a difference:

> God, **Thank you** for the Serenity to accept the things
> I cannot change,
> **Thank you** for the Courage to change the things I can
> And **Thank you** for the Wisdom to know the difference.

Pete was that example of putting the Serenity Prayer into existence. He recognized the need and importance of change. So, using his wisdom and his courage he came up with a better plan and put it into action. Every now and again, we are able to put a bit of serenity, courage, and wisdom into an actionable behavior. When that happens, I think it is important to say thank you.

These virtues—serenity, courage, and wisdom—make a real, and hopefully lasting, positive difference in our lives when challenges arise. Do we learn from our life mistakes? Do we learn from our life triumphs? Do we take time for gratitude when we learn these lessons? When those lessons come to us, it is very important to acknowledge times of courage and wisdom, and to remember to be thankful for those miracles. It is important to recognize that these special gifts are deeply meaningful when we put them into action.

It is all about the plan.

CHAPTER 14

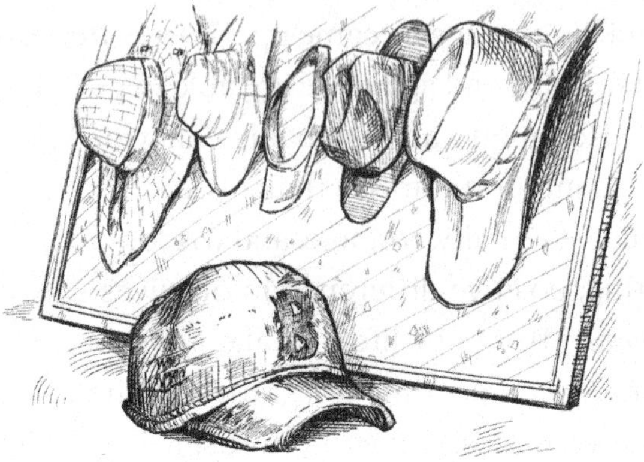

Write Me a Story About Your Hat

The best thing about being a therapist is the opportunity to meet and connect with remarkable people. I truly loved working with a client like Charlie. What a fascinating person. Besides being intelligent and curious, he was uncommonly talented in everything that he put his mind to. It seemed that he made a positive difference in any job or relationship he had. His life reflected his awareness and commitment to making this world a better place, whether he was helping his neighbor with a gardening project, or participating in social change movements. I cannot help but be grateful for how good he was at helping me to be my best so that I could be of better help to him.

Long before we met, Charlie had had an impressive life. As an undergrad, he attended a prestigious university in a vibrant and exciting city that fed his curiosity and grew his capabilities. After graduation, he stayed in that city to take advantage of cultural, social, and vocational opportunities. In that environment, he was able to come to terms with his sexual orientation in a way that would have been very difficult in the small town where he had grown up.

Exploring opportunities, expanding his friendships, and growing his interests and experiences in this fascinating city made this the best time in his life. He was meeting people, enjoying himself, and becoming a young man he could feel good about. He got a job in a career that he loved, including working with colleagues he cherished. He was happy with himself and the way his life was turning out, until an awful traumatic event derailed his sense of trust and safety.

For quite a long time—years, actually—Charlie told no one about what had happened to him. After the traumatic incident, he continued to work hard, make a difference in all of his endeavors, and go on with his life. He stuffed the hurt, the ugliness, and the disruption of the trauma deep inside himself. Outwardly pretending that everything was okay, inwardly, he was falling apart and somewhere inside of him, he knew it. He tried to move ahead with his life and tried to find enjoyment, but he was actually closing himself off from others more and more.

Unable to connect with others as before, Charlie resisted any attempts for closeness, especially from people who wanted to develop a relationship with him on a personal or romantic level.

Emotionally, Charlie was withdrawing to a place deep inside of himself where he lived in shame.

By the time we started to work together, it had been decades since the trauma. He had moved out of his once beloved adopted city closer to his hometown. Back at home in New England, he worked hard for many years in a demanding job, connected as best as he could with his family, and tried to make friends. In actuality, he was pretending all day, every day, that he was fine. However, that deep traumatic wound was continuing to fester and eating up more and more of his emotional energy, hope, and trust.

In time, his life did fall apart as he made excuse after excuse to avoid spending time with family and friends. He would say he had too much work, or he was too tired to attend family functions, answer phone calls, or spend any amount of time with anyone. He stopped doing his laundry, grocery shopping, and other mundane tasks. Things became very dire when he stopped going to work. Cementing himself in a solitary, isolated world, he hoped he would finally disappear and be out of his misery. As the depression progressed, those who knew him were becoming concerned and frightened for his safety.

His family called in the police for a safety check when they were not able to reach him for a number of days. The police found him alone and slowly dying in his home which had become grossly uninhabitable. The heat had been turned off from unpaid bills. There was uneaten food in the kitchen and living room, with unwashed laundry scattered in his bedroom. He had not cleaned any surfaces or the bathroom in quite a while and the house had a very unpleasant smell. Police called an ambulance and he was treated at a nearby hospital for medical care and then was hospitalized at a psychiatric hospital for quite some time.

As a result of the progression of his untreated mental health issues, he lost almost everything—his work, his home, his possessions, his health, his independence. He was at a crossroads in his life. Either he would start to address his trauma, or he would give up completely. Fortunately, he chose to address his trauma.

Charlie was referred to our agency following his hospitalization. After changing therapists a few times, he started to work with me. Entering my office for the first time was a tall, slightly overweight middle-aged man dressed in baggy jeans and a jean jacket wearing fashionable loafers on his feet. Because of a baseball cap pulled tightly over his head it was not easy to see his face. However, once we started to talk, and made some eye contact, I noticed a handsome man with kind brown eyes and a pleasant smile, though there was certainly much sadness and vacancy behind that smile.

Because he had some trepidation about talk therapy, we reviewed what kinds of therapy he had tried. What had worked best? What was not a good fit? It was around the third session that we started to talk about "narrative therapy" which is using writing as a way to connect with the inner person by writing a story about yourself. He had heard about it but had not tried it, so we explored it a bit. He found himself curious and interested in this modality. Charlie loved words and language and writing, sharing with me that over the years writing had always been a helpful and inspiring outlet for him. While talk therapy can be helpful, he knew that he would benefit from an approach that could help him to risk becoming more honest and more transparent. He believed that writing a story about his life could give him a chance to go a little bit deeper, which he longed for more than he realized. We took a chance on using narrative therapy. I was going to come up with the topic and he was going to come up with the story.

When it came time to present the topic, I said to him, "Could you write me a story about your hat? You always have it on when you come to see me. It looks like you have had it for some time. I'll bet there is a story behind that hat." From our first meeting, Charlie wore that hat pulled down as low as he could throughout the session—even when it was quite warm in the office.

"You want me to write a story about my hat?" Looking confused and taking some time he responded, "I don't know. That is not what I was expecting." Pausing again, he considered the request. "But you are right. I have had this hat for a long time. Yeah, I can do that. That might be a good start."

To be honest, Charlie was anticipating that I would ask him to write a story about a troubling parental or personal relationship, or when he first realized he was homosexual, or what led him to pursue the work he had chosen. Writing about his hat was not at all on his mind. Frankly, it wasn't really on my mind either. I trusted my gut on that one. Something inside of me led me to consider a topic that would make him reflect on how even unnoticeable parts of our lives can lead us to some understandings that need to be shared. Out of my mouth came the topic—write me a story about your hat.

He left that session with an assignment. He came back the next week stating that he had started the story but was going to need more time. I told him to take whatever time he needed but I did hope that he would write the story. He continued to come faithfully every week for his sessions. There were a number of other concerns we worked on while the hat story came together. It took a little over a month to complete writing the story about his hat.

The week he came in with the story was unforgettable. He had typed it on his computer and printed it out. The pages were single spaced, paragraph after paragraph, for three pages. He read the story to me, taking his time and allowing for some moments where there needed to be some response. The story was beautifully written. It was so meaningful, touching, and very honest. As the story was shared there were times for some laughter and times where both of us were moved to tears.

The hat he wrote about was a blue Red Sox baseball cap, weathered, frayed, and discolored in some places. The story began with an emphasis on that particular cap. He'd had it for decades, since he was a boy, actually. It reminded him of his father and his uncles who loved the Red Sox. Charlie had special memories of them listening to baseball games on their transistor radio as they played dominoes together. Charlie always wished that he was a better athlete, but that was not his gift. He didn't even really like baseball. But loving his father and his uncles, and wanting to please and connect with them, he would wear that hat.

The next layer of the baseball hat story led to Charlie's young adult years when he was on his own at college and afterwards. Exploring his sexuality was a significant focus in those years and he started to frequent gay bars. Looking for a way to be noticed, he decided he would be the guy in the bar wearing the baseball cap, thinking it gave him an innocent, guy-next-door kind of appeal. And it did. It was often a conversation starter. Many dates happened because of his blue Red Sox baseball cap.

In his written story, he went on to share that he actually became a collector of hats. Over a number of years in his young adulthood, wearing hats became his thing. His collection was interesting and varied. Wearing hats for different moods and occasions and just for fun became an enjoyable activity. What was most fascinating and unexpected was after all these years he still had his hat collection. The only things that he managed to hold onto after losing everything were his hats. He showed me a picture of them. There were dozens of them hung on the wall in his room. They were creatively arranged and looked like an art display decorating his modest little space. He did have a lot of hats!

The other part of his story had to do with shame and hiding. Over time, his Red Sox hat in particular became the hat that he thought he could use to hide from the world in some way. He imagined that if he could hide a part of his face, especially his eyes, maybe people wouldn't see him so much.

There were so many layers of meaning and raw emotion that came from the story of his hat, echoing his life experiences. I was moved beyond words. It opened up a connection between us as he allowed himself some exposure. This was not easy for him to do. I never took it for granted. A sense of safety developed which enhanced our counseling experience. It clearly allowed him to hide less. As a matter of fact, he began to wear a different hat each time he came in for a session. He had not worn those hats in years and he was enjoying wearing them again. It was always a nice conversation starter. He was beginning to enjoy the attention from the receptionists who would regularly comment on his stylish hats. Of more interest was that each hat had a story to tell.

What really happened because of that story is not about hats. It is about the power of telling our story to someone who is really listening. It is such an important gift to be able to give to anyone. After he shared that written story about his hat, Charlie began to share many other stories about his life over the months and years we worked together. He revealed his hurts and traumas. He spoke of missed opportunities for love and committed relationships. He shared about his strengths and triumphs. He explained what made him laugh and feel good. He would tell stories about the present, and many years in the past.

As he opened up, hidden stories of long ago were shared—some humorous, some sad, some just plain awful. It didn't take too much longer after the hat story to share about his unspeakable trauma. In a subdued voice, looking down at the ground, the telling began, "I was so happy before the attack. I was coming home from spending time with friends one evening. Not far from my apartment, someone jumped me. Others joined him and they kept punching, kicking, and hitting me. They were calling me all kinds of vile names. I called out for help and no one responded. They raped me. I was in and out of consciousness a couple of times. Then I was all alone. I somehow made my way back to my apartment and once in, I locked myself in the apartment for a week. Everything inside of me changed after that. Outside of my apartment, I pretended that it didn't happen. But I knew that my spirit and my hope had been broken."

As a result of the rape, he was left with HIV. He shared how he was always so careful about using protection when he had decided to participate in any sexual encounters before the rape. As far as he knew that had been the only time in years when no protection was in use. When he learned about the HIV status, he decided that he was not fit for any close, romantic, or long-term relationships. We took time to acknowledge how difficult it was to share that story as we continued our work to create a space of safety and respect.

The telling of his story had many healing elements. But the real healing is in the relationship that is developed between teller and listener. The therapeutic relationship is different from other relationships because the teller remains the teller and the listener remains the listener. I loved being the listener and witnessing the freeing process of being listened to. There are not many opportunities in life where people are there just for us and we don't have to "share the stage" so to speak. In particular, people who have suffered unspeakable traumas benefit from having someone there, just for them. It helps them to get some of that story told, and some of that hurt healed a little bit.

Charlie had always been a curious and logical person. He had many difficult personal and metaphysical questions about the trauma that upended his life. He wondered why it had happened to him. Had he done something to deserve it? Was there something wrong with him because he was born homosexual? What will it take for bigotry and intolerance to come to an end? He knew that he was a good person who was caring and generous with others all of his life. These questions mattered much to Charlie as he struggled finding answers. Platitudes were unhelpful, so we sat with the ambiguity and pain of not having answers to many of his difficult and emotional questions.

Who knows why Charlie was dealt the hand in life he had been given? He didn't know. I certainly did not. Life seemed to be unfair for so many of the people I came in contact with in the mental health work I did. Why do some people end up in poverty, or burdened with mental illness, or the victims of senseless and cruel trauma?

Some of it is systemic, built into societal and cultural norms. That in itself is stupid and unfair to me. Perhaps society can find more effective strategies and policies to address the injustices of poverty, racism, sexism, etc. However, the fact remains that some people just get dealt horrible life experiences that are not systemic, and are not a result of bad decisions, or race, or poverty, or culture. I had the privilege throughout my work to accompany my clients on a life journey that was difficult and exhausting for them. They did not deserve the amount of suffering their lives entailed. These incredibly brave souls continued to live their lives as best as they could. They found reasons to rejoice when possible. They allowed themselves moments of complaint as well. I suppose there are times when that is the best that most of us can do.

It may be a reflection of the story of Job in the Old Testament. In the book of Job, "an upright man," he loses his possessions, his children, and his wealth and prestige. His friends lament with him on his horrible trauma. They tell him it is because he has sinned. His friends tell him that he has offended God in some way. He needs to repent so that God will take away the "punishments" laid upon him. Job protested to his friends and to God that he had done nothing that would explain the bad turn in his life. To him, there was no reason for the calamities he was suffering. The end of the book of Job is a conversation between Job and God about suffering.

There really is no explanation from God for the suffering that Job underwent. God points out that people just don't know what they don't know. God reveals to Job God's omnipotence. In the face of that reality, Job is humbled. Being faced with the omnipotence of God reminded Job that he does not know, nor is he able to fathom the mind of God. In his humility, Job accepts that trusting God and relying on faith is his response to what he does not and cannot understand.

While I continue to be bothered about so much suffering, I also continue to work on coming to terms with the truth that I lack comprehension about suffering as well. I am trying to come to terms with what it means when it is said "It is what it is." While this is true, it is not an easy truth. It is a truth that hurts, actually.

In the end, there was so little that I could do to help Charlie with the reality of his challenges and sufferings, except to listen, to support and to be there in my caring way. Charlie struggled with his life story until the end. It was difficult to reconcile a life that continued to be unrecognizable to him. He was a good man who always felt like he had failed and lost sight of the person he had hoped to be.

Charlie died while we were still working together. He had medical challenges in addition to his HIV status that ran their course and his time on earth came to its end. It took me a couple weeks to put someone else in Charlie's counseling spot. I needed to make an adjustment. I needed some time to go through some grieving and to give myself time to say goodbye in the way that worked best for me. There will always be a special place in my heart for the guy who wrote me the story about his hat. The power of one's story is amazing. Somehow both of us were changed for good because of that story. I hope and pray that all of us have an opportunity to share our stories. You never know what layers of truth and healing somehow make their way into the telling of our stories.

CHAPTER 15

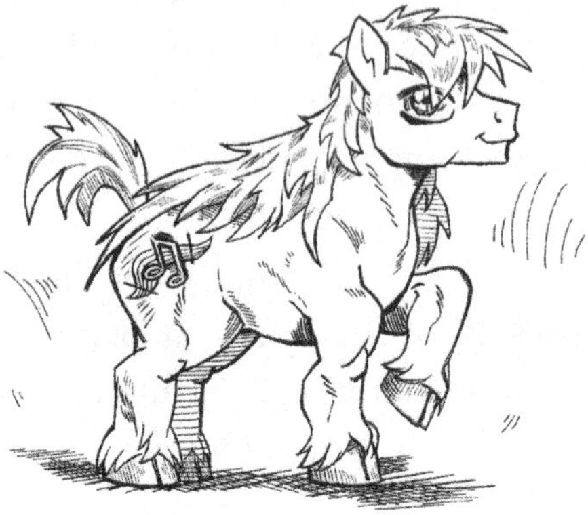

Manifestations

How fortunate for me that in my last two years of work as a therapist, I got to meet and work with David. His state social worker referred him for mental health counseling because he was just about impossible to live with. As such, any opportunity for independent living was not going to happen without some changes.

Born with cerebral palsy, and exhibiting autistic behaviors as well, David made daily life chaotic and challenging. Some serious conflicts had developed with his second adult foster home placement. It was reported that David had frequent anger outbursts. He was at times belligerent, and regularly uncooperative. His hygiene was atrocious. He rarely showered or washed his clothing. He hated brushing his teeth, resulting in foul smelling breath and tooth decay. To make things even worse, he regularly sang and played musical instruments in the home, ignoring the time of day and volume of his "performances."

David was in his mid-twenties when we started to work together. Over six feet tall, his long lanky limbs hanging uncomfortably by his side, David was a noticeable figure. With bushy, unruly dark brown hair, and a ready and easy smile, David's eyes were either focused on me with intensity or they were darting all over the place. He was very talkative and articulate. His imagination was boundless.

He was fascinated with music; it was amazing how many instruments he could play, including the acoustic and electric guitar, bass, harmonica, penny whistle, and a number of other unusual stringed instruments. He actually played some with proficiency. He was completely self-taught although he would say that YouTube was his music teacher. A prolific songwriter, it was not unusual for him to write multiple songs in one day. Some of them were very primitive but others were really quite good. He was especially fond of folk music and had a fascination with folk singers from the 1960s and 1970s. Fortune put him in the life of a caring older couple who adopted him when he was a young boy. "They were hippies," David declared with much pride and gratitude as they had introduced him to Pete Seeger; Phil Ochs; Peter, Paul and Mary; and a number of other folk and protest singers of that time. This music became a major influence, as his current songs reflected. As we got to know each other, his ability to articulate his understanding of some rather complex political and social history made it very interesting to talk with him.

His adoptive mother had passed away when he was in his late teens. He missed her tremendously. He and his adoptive father were not getting along very well. Within a short time after his adoptive mother had died his father petitioned to put him into state care. David had been receiving services through the state department of developmental disabilities throughout his life. As a result of his troublesome issues with his adoptive father, he was placed in an adolescent group home for people with developmental disabilities. As a young adult he had started to participate in housing opportunities using adult foster homes. He was now in his second adult foster home.

When we first started working together, David would downplay his behaviors surrounding his living situation. He did admit that he was having difficulties with his housemate and did not dispute the complaints leveled against him. He just did not want to make any changes in his behaviors regarding this situation. He wanted the stress that went with these issues to just go away. After all, he was a peaceful person who just wanted a world of justice and love.

Well, David was asked to leave the foster home where he was staying. He was going to be moving to a group home for developmentally disabled adults. Of the ten people living there, only one or two of them were verbal. None were as verbal or as capable as David. This change in his living situation left him feeling depressed and discouraged. There was one staff person who did connect with David but that person worked only part time. David got some needed time and attention from this staff person and his hygiene did improve, but it was not consistent.

In addition to his love of music and his prolific creativity as a songwriter, David also talked regularly about his "manifestations." I have to admit, this approach to managing stress was new to me and I wanted to learn about it. Luckily, David was a good teacher. He would take the time to explain to me what his manifestations meant to him and how much he relied on them. His manifestations centered around a fascination with *My Little Pony.*

I learned that manifestation to Gen Xers is an approach to getting something that you want by using a type of positive thinking. David believed that if he thought hard enough and believed completely enough, he could will his desires and wishes into being. Hence, he spent much time imagining and thinking about being something other than what he was and somewhere other than where he was.

On our second appointment, David introduced me to his favorite *My Little Pony* animated characters. *My Little Pony* was an animated series on television from the 1980s that was generally geared to children ages six to eleven. He would spend much time on YouTube or on the My Little Pony website watching animations and studying the numerous characters who helped others and offered their friendship. He shared that he was, in fact, manifesting into one of these particular animated characters. He asked if I knew anything about that character. I had to admit that I did not but I would be interested in learning more about the character if that was important to him.

He went on to explain that he was, in fact, becoming that character. When I asked what that meant he explained he was actually turning blue, growing a mane and a tail and well-developed muscles just like his favorite *My Little Pony* character. He hoped that maybe in a month or so, he would actually be that character. That is what he meant by his manifestations. While this description of his words and thoughts sound a bit psychotic, it never seemed to approach the clinical status that David was out of touch with reality. He was much involved in his real life as he described in detail the happenings of his day. Articulating his displeasure with a housemate or what took place at his day program, David was totally in touch with the reality of his life.

While it sometimes sounded like David was psychotic, it seemed more likely that he had developed a coping mechanism for his stress and sadness that involved what he was calling "manifestations." It was an escape for him from the sadness and impossibility of his current life circumstances. It became clear to me that David used his wishes and imagination to find momentary escapes from the lonely and frustrating reality of his everyday life. He was stuck in a living situation that was not healthy for him. If he were going to achieve a more independent life, there was change that needed to happen. However, the change that was needed did not involve turning into a life-size blue pony.

I asked for more information about what kind of personality his animated character had. David explained that his character was peaceful but strong, a leader of the pack and someone who loved himself. We talked about what important qualities those are in an animated character as well as in a person. There was agreement between us that David could use the positive personal qualities of his favorite animated character(s) to make meaningful and achievable changes in his life. He couldn't wait to introduce me to all of the animated characters that he loved.

It was going to take a lot more exploration and much more discussion. I am not very tech savvy. Finding and exploring websites can be a challenge for me. I was going to have to learn to be more in the know if I was going to learn about animated *My Little Pony*. What I learned quite quickly is that *My Little Pony* is a "thing." For reasons unknown to me, millions of people, adults and children the world over, seem to have a fascination with *My Little Pony* animated characters. There are dozens of them. They run the gamut of the cute little ponies I remember from the cartoon, to the more anime looking characters of today. Some of the newer characters are rather scary looking.

Every time we had a session I would ask about his manifestations and he would talk about his favorite characters. It was one of the ways that we could explore what he was drawn to in them. What qualities and behaviors were catching his imagination? I was hoping that maybe we could use that information to help David change some of his more unpleasant behaviors. His wishes regarding his manifestations focused on love, beauty, and finding happiness, connection, and freedom. We did make use of those themes during sessions with the hopes that he could manifest them into some positive and helpful habits and behaviors.

David and I sought out a number of different approaches to address the behaviors, or lack thereof, that were holding him back from more independent living opportunities. One approach that I had grown fond of started with my earlier work on mobile treatment teams. We would accompany clients into the community for normal everyday experiences. I started to meet with David at the end of my workday a couple of times a month. We would go for a car ride or go for a walk. Once in a while we stopped for a hamburger at a very affordable local restaurant that offered table service. I benefited from observing David in social situations and it also helped to connect us in more meaningful ways. The first time we went for a hamburger was quite informative for me. David was paying close attention to how I interacted with the wait staff and he would copy my behaviors in his own way, smiling at the wait staff and ordering his meal just the way I had done.

David always had much to say. We never struggled with a topic to discuss that addressed approaches to making changes that would improve his chances for more independent living. He was so interesting to me. However, as much as we both enjoyed our sessions together, he was not making much progress when it came to personal responsibility for hygiene and self-care.

As it so happened at one of our hamburger outings, not too long before my retirement, David was once again introducing me to a *My Little Pony* character that he was "manifesting" into. He showed me the character on his smartphone. The character was a beautiful, strong looking adult pony with a long glorious mane and muscular legs. I commented to David how handsome this pony was. I then asked David, "How do you think he got his mane to be so beautiful?" David shared his ideas quite readily, talking about shampooing and caring for his mane. I then commented to David that he also had very nice hair. I asked him what it would take for his hair to look like his new favorite character's. We had a lengthy talk about caring for hair using shampoo and conditioner and how to make sure that it is done regularly in a shower so he could keep all of his body looking like his favorite character. David decided on a plan to make this happen. We determined that when we met again in a couple of weeks, he was going to let me know how he made out.

Two weeks passed and I met him at his group home. We had planned to go for a walk on that beautiful spring afternoon. David was waiting for me on the sidewalk outside. As I got out of the car he exclaimed excitedly, "Celeste, look at my hair!!" I commented on how good his hair looked. It did look really good. "Smell me," he said with gusto. "I smell like birthday cake!" as he extended his right arm for me to take a whiff.

"How did you manage all this?" I asked.

He told me all about his new routines and efforts at better and more consistent hygiene. As we walked, we reviewed his achievements and current success. He shared how good it felt to "manifest" something that other people could see and experience at the same time he experienced it. We stopped for a few minutes to sit at a nearby eatery for an iced tea and he shared his newest song with me. The lyrics used the imagery of finding something precious within a deep well. It was quite a moving piece.

On our way back to his home, David did something that he had not done before. He asked me about me. He started his questions stating that we had been meeting for almost two years and he didn't know anything about me. Knowing that I would be retiring soon, he asked what I was planning to do with my retirement. He asked if I had children, and what hobbies and interests I had. It was sweet and endearing. I answered his questions honestly and I hope sufficiently. I was never comfortable sharing personal information about myself with clients, but in this simple encounter it did feel like the right thing to do.

That was one of our last counseling sessions together. I was very moved by the entirety of that appointment. Somehow, we began to "manifest" a way for each of us to connect with a bit of our truest selves that last hour and a half or so that we spent walking and talking over an iced tea. For many it may not have looked like a therapy session, but for the both of us it was one of the best sessions that we had over those many encounters.

I learned some very valuable lessons from David. His preoccupation with manifestations was much more important than I realized. Manifestations have to do with meaningful exposure, expression and revelation. I lost sight many times over the years about how I express and reveal myself. I was taught in graduate school that part of the work of a therapist is to be a mirror to the client so that the client can focus on themselves and their healing. We are expected to keep ourselves mostly out of the conversation. For the most part, that was how I did my work. I was not one to reveal much about myself within my counseling relationships except for very general information that most of the time did not reveal much of anything at all. Frankly, I believe that was the right approach for more sessions than not.

But every now and again, exposing and revealing oneself provided a connection with a person that truly enhanced the counseling experience. I think the timing when David asked me about me was not at all an accident. It seemed that David began to discover what manifesting is about for him. I think at that appointment, part of him was realizing that manifestation was about how to connect with the world and the people in it. He had been using his preoccupation with his animated characters as a way to escape and avoid his loneliness and sadness. He wasn't sure how to connect to the world and the people in it. However, something changed in him. As he connected more authentically with himself, he wanted to connect with another human being—me. His song revealed that he had found something precious deep within himself. It was time to manifest that precious person to another human being. It was time to risk connecting with another person by making space within himself for someone else.

I realize as I write this story that counseling and therapy is all about making room for another person within yourself. It is always about revealing something about yourself to another human being, so that what is holding us back in life can be better understood. Manifesting our deepest hurts and longings with the intention of finding healing and connection is the best of what can happen in therapy and within relationships. I have no doubt that David continued to be enamored with *My Little Pony*. Although I never quite understood the fascination, he helped me appreciate and respect how important it is to consider and name what we want to manifest to the world when it comes to who we are...and who we are becoming.

CHAPTER 16

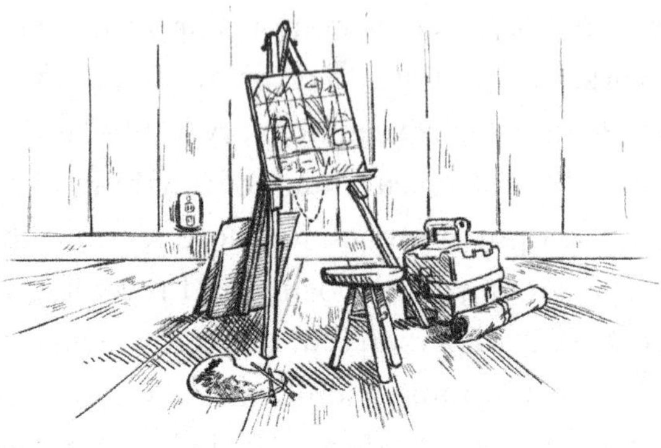

Funny Bones

I had the privilege and blessing to work with Sophie as her therapist for six years. Because we had the benefit of time, I was able to accompany Sophie on an incredible journey of healing and discovery.

Entering my office for that first appointment was an attractive woman in her thirties with long, curly brown hair, dressed in black leggings and a flowing blouse with purple, blue, and white flowers. Holding back her long hair on the right side was a purple sparkly butterfly hairclip. Her purple plastic-rimmed eyeglasses begin to fog up and she cries and explains that she is seeking counseling because someone very close to her died recently. Her mother had died of a drug overdose the month before, leaving Sophie devastated over this sudden, unexpected loss.

The loss of a parent, child, family member, life partner, or dear friend because of a drug overdose is so very, very painful. The emotional toll is overwhelming. Sophie had to work through hundreds of thoughts, memories, emotions and experiences as she trudged through her grief. I sat with Sophie session after session, feeling as if

I were emotionally holding onto her to save her from being drowned by grief, anger, confusion, and dozens of other emotions. It was quite emotional for both of us, especially in the early months of treatment.

Sophie presented as a person in deep emotional pain. She was sad, confused, overwhelmed, angry, lost, heartbroken, inconsolable. When I started working with Sophie, she spent months crying throughout her sessions. For many weeks, months, and years, she needed a safe place to cry and emote. She just needed to be in her place of pain without judgment, without having to "get over it." So rather than "getting over it," we went through it, together, as best as we could.

Sophie was suffering from what is termed *complicated grief*. A common understanding of this diagnosis involves grief that is difficult to resolve because it involves trauma. It is associated with substantial impairment in work, health, and social functioning. Grief left Sophie unable to connect with family and friends in a healthy way. It hurt her tremendously that her other family members were not as grieved as she was. As she lamented about that belief it led to more pain and isolation. She was unable to work and many days she could barely get out of bed, never mind out of the house. She would have outbursts of anger which made it difficult for her to participate in social situations. She believed that people were thinking ill of her. It was not unusual for her to interpret any number of conversations, interactions, or text messages as critical of her or, at the least, insensitive to her grief. She would talk about coming across a person who may have supplied drugs to her mother which led her to any number of emotional responses. She was not able to contain her anger when this happened. Unable to manage these thoughts and feelings, at times, it was unsafe for her to be out shopping, or sitting in a waiting room, or driving down an unfamiliar street.

There is no timeline, no blueprint, no step-by-step process to follow. Grief work is a singular, individual experience. We started with baby steps as we began the work to help her through her grief process. She cried. She spoke when she was ready. She worked on finding a pathway to remember her mother in healthy ways as she told story after story about their complicated relationship. We talked about safety and about finding ways to work through her thoughts, emotions, and reactions in safe and helpful ways. Sometimes, as a therapist, you need to follow a client into a painful place—into that deep dark hole and through the seemingly endless tunnel of grief. While there, the therapist does their best to light an emotional candle of support and understanding. I found myself demonstrating as best as I could that Sophie was not alone, that she was loved and being looked after not only by me, but by her many other supports, and we both believed, somehow, by her mother.

It was impressive how Sophie sought out others who were going through what she was going through. She had always been very adept at managing social media and she found online support groups of others who had also lost family members to a drug overdose. She would spend hours online communicating with people who were experiencing what she was experiencing. This online community provided a forum to share her pain, ask questions and, in time, offer support to others in similar pain. She participated in public gatherings with other people who were going through the same thing. She went to a number of International Overdose Awareness Days at the state house. There she would stand up with dozens of other families who were going through the same experience. They were there to ask for help to address this horrible public health problem.

As we worked together over weeks and months, Sophie would often express her hurt and frustration about her mother's years of drug use and addiction. She had only known her mother as a drug addict. Sophie would cry and ask, "Why couldn't she stop?" "Why did she keep on using when she would tell me over and over again that she was sober and that she had stopped using?" "She loved her drugs more than she loved me—I know it!" The reality of any person who is in a close relationship with anyone who is struggling with addiction is that the relationship is confusing, frustrating, and painful. Sophie did experience her mother as someone who lied to her and hid drug use from her. Over the years, her mother participated in numerous treatment programs followed by periods of sobriety and, unfortunately, repeated relapses. Sophie found the relationship exhausting.

One session as Sophie was continuing to work through her anger about her mother's addictive behaviors, we started to talk about things that Sophie, herself, had a hard time resisting. "Well—I really like Funny Bones," she said. She shared how there were many days that she just could not resist eating a Funny Bone cupcake or two and sometimes three at a sitting. She explained that as she was going through this most difficult time, she was indulging quite a bit.

Before I could stop myself, I heard myself responding "I love Funny Bones too! What's not to love?" We shared our favorite things about Funny Bones—a chocolate cupcake with a creamy peanut butter filling surrounded by milk chocolate. Add a nice cold glass of milk—yum! Then we sort of stopped and noticed that we were getting all gushy over Funny Bones cupcakes and we started to giggle a bit, which soon became a good laugh.

Much of therapy is serious and difficult, there is no doubt about that. However, when you share that first laugh and that moment of just silly indulgence, a different kind of healing can begin. It is the crack that lets the light in.

As silly as this moment was, it became a breakthrough moment. I shared with her that if we cannot resist a Funny Bone, we can't even imagine what her mother was experiencing with an addiction to crack cocaine. Her mother's preoccupation was at least ten thousand times more difficult to resist than our obsession with Funny Bones. We talked about how her mother was constantly having to resist the games her brain would play on her. In Alcoholics Anonymous, they call addiction a hijacking of the brain. This describes what seems to be going on. Her brain never stopped making excuses for reasons to use the drug. The inner brain chatter was continuous for her mother: "Just this one time," "No one is going to know," "You're just having a good time with friends and you didn't even have to pay for it," "I had a tough day and just needed a break," "I had a good day and just needed to celebrate."

We talked about how addiction is really not about willpower or intelligence or love. The addict's brain tells them that something is important when it is not. It is a terrible condition that lays horrible burdens on individuals, families, and communities.

We absolutely needed to work on this part of her healing process. Addiction is awful! I would not wish that condition on anyone. I fantasize about the day that science will provide more answers about how addiction works and, more importantly, how to help the brain resist addictive tendencies. Someday we will be able to prevent the kind of intoxication that leads to addiction. Humans have been fascinated with alteration of the brain for millennia. We seek out ways to escape reality and alter our human experiences by thinking that we are having a great time when we are intoxicated. Most of us will not get hooked and addicted. But for those who do, it is a sorry and painful life experience.

Every now and again, when Sophie began to complain about her mother and addiction or about other people and their faults, we would look at each other and one or the other of us would say "Funny Bones." That was our cue that we were obsessing about something that led us away from our healing path and towards unfair judgement and needless anger. That catch word became one of those helpful tools for redirection. We all have those times in our lives when we need a little redirection. In our work as therapists, we help clients appreciate the importance of knowing when and how to redirect those thoughts that tend to bring us or others harm. For Sophie and I, our Funny Bones cue was an easy, helpful reminder to not take ourselves more seriously than we need to.

Sophie and I talked for hours and hours about addiction. She had to come to terms with her own patterns of addictive behavior.

There appeared to be a family pattern of addiction through multiple generations in Sophie's family and on both sides of her family. She worked hard to identify those patterns and to come up with a plan for herself that led to a safer, more honest life. Surprisingly, she came upon a new path that became an amazing healing journey.

What is so incredible about Sophie's healing journey is that she found her way to a most wonderful and positive path. Five months or so after her mother passed, she began to paint. Her mother had been an artist. Sophie did not grow up doing much art because she was trying not to be like her mother. She appreciated that her mother did have artistic talent but she also thought her mother was a bit odd. After her mother died, Sophie gathered as many of her mother's possessions as she could and kept them in her apartment. It was a way for her to feel that somehow her mother was still around. Most of those possessions were blank canvases, paintbrushes, and paints. Out of boredom or curiosity or perhaps something else, she picked up her mother's art supplies and started looking through YouTube videos to teach herself how to paint. And lo and behold, Sophie discovered that she really liked painting. She found herself watching more YouTube videos to learn and try new techniques. She discovered that she was very creative and had a natural talent for painting—much like her mother. She would often lose track of time as she worked on her canvases. As she continued to experience this wonderful connection with her mother, she also developed a healing connection with herself.

As Sophie continued to heal, she also began to open herself up in so many remarkable ways. About a year into our counseling sessions, she began to share her art with others. She started by reaching out to senior living places and offering a monthly art group at several local assisted living residences. Another year or so after, she also started to offer "paint nights" at various locations, discovering that she was good at sharing art. She used this experience to share about her own healing journey by talking about how she lost her mother to addiction and in many ways lost part of herself as well. She acknowledged that painting and sharing art had become how she also found a path to healing, a path to her more authentic self, and a path to a happiness she had never known before.

As in all journeys there are ups and downs. Sophie had a bumpy ride ahead of her. She used her therapy sessions to work through the bumps and to consider adjustments in her approaches and assumptions. As it turned out, Sophie is quite hilarious. She loves to laugh and to tell stories about her life's adventures. Early in therapy Sophie could spend almost an entire session crying and complaining about the faults and failings of others. Complaining about others is actually a very popular defense mechanism for most of us. As the artwork and healing continued, her "complaints" became stories of the ridiculous nature of all of us. She was as much a comedian as she was an artist. We laughed a lot the last few years of therapy.

One of the lessons Sofie taught me is quite profound. She noticed as she learned more about painting and doing art that there is an ugly phase in the painting process. In the earlier phases of painting, the painting looks quite awful, she stated. She explained that as an artist you have an idea of where you want to get to with your painting but it is a process that takes time, diligence, and persistence. If you give up before you get through the ugly phase (the unfinished part of the painting process) you will miss out on getting to your work of art. One session Sophie shared that her healing journey also had ugly phases. She learned that while she wanted to give up and believe that life was just ugly, in fact, it was not. She had learned that persisting was part of the healing process. The only way out is through. Because she kept coming to treatment, kept seeking her path for healing, kept connecting with healing allies, she was getting healthier. She was laughing, connecting, sharing, and inviting others to be a part of their own healing journey. What an amazing person she turned out to be!

What incredible lessons she taught me. Persistence and vision are crucial to our healing. Making connections with our own creativity to reach deeper and produce more lasting change is also so important in the healing process. In addition, sharing and connecting with others about our journeys, in respectful, interesting, and enjoyable ways cannot be underestimated.

When it came time for me to retire and for Sophie to seek out another therapist to continue her work, we talked about how we could remember each other in a special way. We decided that each time we had a Funny Bone we would say a prayer for each other. We would keep in mind that that little indulgence was a way to remember that we had grown together, learned much from each other, and had developed a love for each other that was special and lasting. So, as I feast on a Funny Bone I offer "Here's to you Sophie. May life continue to be a fascinating, loving, and creative healing journey for you."

CHAPTER 17

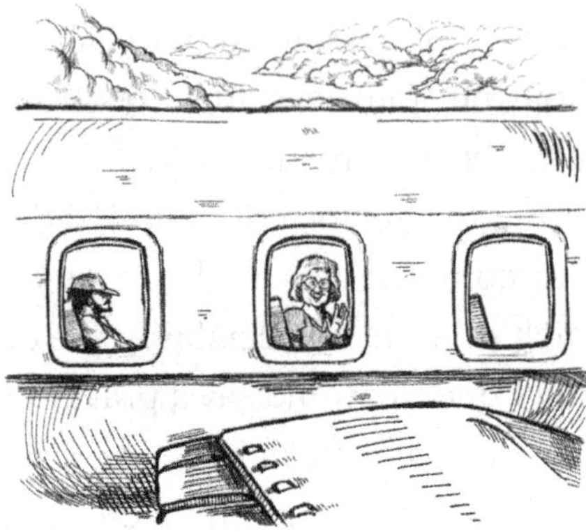

Book Your Flight

Do you have a patron saint? If you do, I bet you have many things for which to be grateful. A patron saint is a very good thing to have. Your patron saint is an intercessor to the God in whom you believe. They do not take the place of God and they are not divine beings. Patron saints are simply persons of faith who lived lives that made a significant difference in the time in which they lived. Or they are persons who had exemplary faith and were willing to die for what they believed.

Patron saints are very popular and of much significance in the faith I was raised in. Churches, hospitals, universities, and other community buildings are named in honor of saints. Countries all over the world have patron saints, as do hundreds of professions and persons with all kinds of conditions. Some examples of those with patron saints are bricklayers (St. Stephen) and candlemakers (St. Ambrose), doctors (St. Luke), lawyers (SS. Genesius and Thomas More), and accountants (St. Matthew). Patron saints are also called upon to help with certain conditions like throat trouble (SS. Cecilia and Blaise), ulcers (St. Charles), cancer (St. Peregrine), and even cramps (St. Maurice). There also seems to be a patron saint for cranky children! (St. Sebastian)

Early on in my career, one of my female clients introduced me to her patron saint. She came in for her session one day and said, "Do you know who St. Dymphna is?" I responded that I did not. She then produced a prayer card with St. Dymphna's picture on one side and a prayer on the other that indicated that St. Dymphna was the patron saint of those suffering with nervous and mental afflictions. My client was pretty sure that St. Dymphna was helping her. She talked about her devotion to the saint as she had a practice that included a prayer to the saint every day for help and intervention. The prayer card of St. Dymphna she brought that day was for me to have. She wanted to share her hope with me. I hung the card on my bulletin board and I have to admit, it reminded me to say a little prayer for my clients and for myself regularly.

I learned what I could about the patron saint of persons with mental afflictions. It is quite a tragic story actually. Dymphna was born in Ireland in the seventh century to a pagan Irish king and his Christian wife. The queen died at a young age, and left her husband bereft. He was inconsolable and it is said that his grief pushed him to the verge of mental collapse. He wanted a wife that would be exactly like his first queen. As life would have it, his young teenage daughter was a spitting image of her mother, his deceased queen. His advisors encouraged him to marry his daughter and put himself out of his misery. She adamantly refused his request. The king went into a fury. Her confessor, Father Gerbern, supported her refusal and was very concerned about her safety now that she had denied her father. Dymphna fled with the priest and her two trusted servants. They found themselves in the city of Antwerp, on the coast of Belgium. They ended up settling in the nearby village of Geel.

Legend states that while living in Geel, Dymphna built a hospital for the poor and sick and those with mental issues. However, in using her wealth to build the hospital, it made it easier for her father to locate her. Her father set out to bring her back to Ireland and to force her to marry him. He found her and her small entourage in Geel. She again refused him. In his blind anger he killed her by using his own sword to cut off her head. She was just a teenager. Because of her horrible death and as a tribute to her strength in maintaining her dignity, she was revered by the townspeople where she was killed. She was named as a martyr for her faith and eventually canonized.

Legends abound that those persons with mental illness who witnessed her death were instantly cured. As time went on, a church was eventually built around the place of her death. Stories began to circulate that persons with mental illness were experiencing relief from their troubles at the site. By 1480 so many pilgrims were arriving in need of treatment for mental illnesses that the church was expanded and a hospital was added. In 1532 a larger church and shrine to St. Dymphna was erected and still stands today over her burial site in the city of Geel in Belgium.

I am all in favor of anything that can bring a little hope. Having a bit of a change in perspective and maybe a little bit of belief that there is someone bigger than us provides us with spiritual tools that can become part of the healing process. It is not easy to hang onto hope day after day. I heard so many stories from clients over the years reflecting burdens and sufferings that were staggering. It would seem like the light around them was dulled, or missing. It felt like I was walking through some of those dark spaces with my clients.

It was during those moments when I could get lost in the darkness as well. Sometimes it would feel overwhelming and I would find myself emotionally creating some distance between myself and my clients. Even though I had been trained to focus on techniques, approaches, and skills to help clients through those times, I am not sure that I was always that helpful for them. There were times over the years I would begin to question and doubt myself. I would begin to think that I was not at all cut out for the work I had chosen.

Of course, doubt and insecurity are not unusual in anyone's life, but I would begin to feel that it was not fair to clients if I was becoming unable to provide support, presence, and help that was beneficial to them. I fantasized about any number of other jobs that would probably be a better fit for me like selling plants, or decluttering, or working as a bookkeeper. I wondered if I would be better off not working with people at all. I am not totally sure how I made it through those times and moments. But I did. I just kept showing up. Most of what is called for in the healing journey is that we just keep showing up for the life we are given.

I would get myself to work day after day, and I would look at that prayer card and say the prayer on the back of the card. I think it did help. It was a continual reminder to me that I could not do this work on my own, by myself. My faith and my faith experience supported the hope that led me through the years of my work. One of the images that is used in my faith tradition when talking about saints is "a cloud of witnesses." I love that image: a cloud of witnesses. Imagine that there is this spiritual resource of a healthy and loving energy of support, advocacy, listening, guidance, and presence. For me, saints reminded me to stay open to what is possible and to point me toward what is light, healing, and good. Saints also reminded me that it is my responsibility to see light in others, especially when things seem so difficult, cloudy, or dark.

It seemed that when I was feeling most discouraged about myself and my work, I would have an encounter with a client that would reassure me that what I was doing mattered. Clients were responding, and in many cases were making some progress in the course of their challenging lives. They also would keep coming. They trusted me and they trusted in the process. My experience of continuing in this chosen vocation for as long as I did confirmed that I was never alone in the work and, in fact, the work belonged to something bigger than me. The experience of trusting in a loving presence, and trying to get out of the way so that love could do what it needed to do, made it possible for me to stay in the work for decades. That was the lesson over and over again: get out of the way and let the healing happen. Just as there is a cloud of witnesses in the saints, much of the work I was participating in involved witnessing and accompanying clients in their mental health journeys. While there were skills and techniques that I could pass on, much of what I did involved supporting, encouraging, and cheering clients on to a better life experience, one they could claim as their own.

Thankfully I was also blessed to have a number of good and caring supervisors over the years. I had my own support system to help keep me afloat when I most needed help. People who showed up for me the way I showed up for my clients. Making time for my own therapy over the years also provided that bit of perspective that is so crucial in being available for others.

I learned over the years to pay attention to the little things in life. For me it was making time for the things that kept me healthy enough that I could keep showing up for the work. In addition to connecting to what I believe in every day, and keeping connected with my own support system, I also made it a point to find time for a "treat" on a regular basis. For me, it's often chocolate. In my office I would keep a little basket on my desk with individually wrapped little Dove chocolates. It was a nice way to connect with clients and many of them appreciated the gesture. We would share our stories about how much chocolate was a comfort. In addition, the little individual Dove chocolates have a saying in the wrapper. They were often a source of small inspirations. Every now and again, the saying contributed to part of our conversation during our treatment sessions. Sometimes they seemed to fit what was going on for a client on a given day. I was always a bit amazed when that would happen.

Wouldn't you know it, as I began my last month of work before my retirement, I opened up a Dove chocolate and the saying for the first week of that month was "You've got this." I was quite pleased by the saying and hung it on my bulletin board to remind me that all was going to work out as it should. A couple weeks later, my Dove chocolate wrapper message was "Book your flight." I must admit that the saying blew me away. For years I had been squirreling away a bit of my money planning a visit to Europe after I retired. I wanted to go to Belgium to visit St. Dymphna's shrine to say thank you. What are the chances that my Dove chocolate would provide confirmation that getting over to Belgium was something that needed to happen? The universe works in strange ways indeed.

A few months after I retired, I flew to Belgium and visited the Church of St. Dymphna in Geel. It was a most beautiful and moving experience. At first, I was the only person there on that particular afternoon. I used that time alone for some personal reflection and prayer. A little while after that, the parishioner who was there to greet pilgrims that day arrived. I introduced myself to Jan and told him that I had come from the United States to say thank you to St. Dymphna who had become my patron saint. I shared with him that I had worked in the mental health field for decades and how it seemed that my reaching out to her had made a difference. I was thankful for her support through the years. He was so gracious and appreciative of my story. He spent almost two hours walking me through the church. He pointed out the significance of each stained-glass window, side altars, paintings, and other works of art. He walked me to the part of the church that centuries ago had been a part of the hospital for mentally ill patients. He updated me on how his town had become a center of treatment for the mentally ill over the decades. Jan shared that Geel is now one of the best places in Europe to get mental health treatment. It was such a wonderful experience for me. I am so grateful that I had the opportunity to visit the church and most importantly to say thank you.

In the last few years of my work, I often found myself reflecting on gratitude. The more years I spent in the work, the more it became apparent that it was a privilege to be a part of someone's healing journey. It also was very clear that I was always a part of something bigger than myself.

During the Covid pandemic, when everything shut down and there was no place to go, I came across Mat and Savanna Shaw on YouTube. They are a daddy/daughter singing duo from Utah. I listened to them every day for months. I so enjoyed their singing and the sweet relationship they shared. It was a comfort in a difficult and confusing time. One of the songs they sang that I was especially drawn to was "Thankful" by Sager, Foster, and Page. I played it every day for over a year. It became a part of my daily prayer and I continue to listen to the song often.

Here is the verse from "Thankful" that reminds me about faith and what saints are about:

> *"Even with our differences, there is a place we're all connected; each of us can find each other's light . . . It's up to us to be the change and even though this world needs so much more, there's so much to be thankful for."*

I am so grateful for being a part of the journeys of so many wonderful people. Through dark times and into times of more light and growth, I grew and experienced so many valuable life lessons because of the fascinating people I had the blessing to get to know over the years, clients and colleagues alike. It seems that we all benefited from being able to tell and listen to the stories of lives as they are being lived.

Music has been another source of support and healing throughout my life. My first paid work in the mental health field was at the agency called CHAOS. That experience left me with the song "Leaving Things in CHAOS." That song was a reminder to me over the years to let the work be what it needed to be. I was not the one in control of anyone's healing journey. My role was to accompany, support, and witness how healing happens in our lives. It is also no surprise that the song that accompanied me through the last couple years of my work in the mental health field was "Thankful." That is the theme that reverberated through me for months as my work journey came to its close.

I guess no matter how chaotic things appeared at times over the years, a little bit of chocolate, a patron saint, helpful songs and caring family, colleagues, and friends seemed to be just the ingredients I needed to teach me the lessons I needed to learn. How else would I have survived to tell the tale of this worthwhile adventure?

As I came to the end of this incredible and unexpected journey, my heart, mind, and soul were feeling so very THANKFUL.

For friends, colleagues, and staff at the Community Care Alliance in Woonsocket, RI. So grateful for your guidance, support, and caring over the years.
God bless you all.

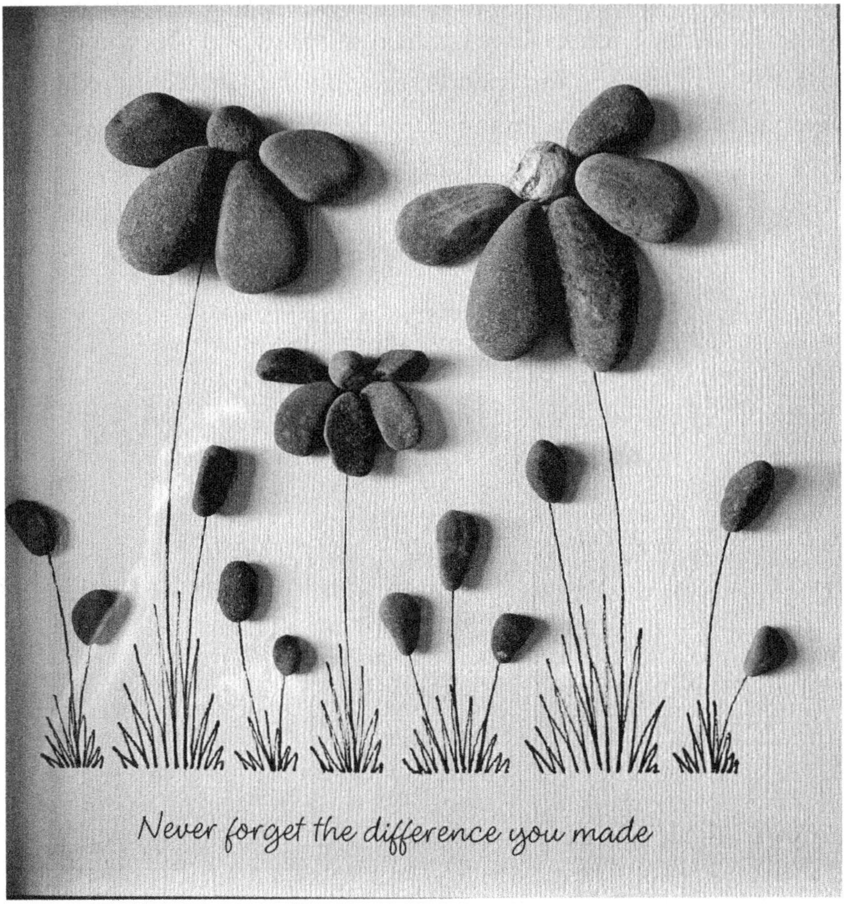

Pebble art by Sarah Hough
Sarah's Craft Chest https://sarahscraftchest.etsy.com/

(This lovely piece of art was given to me by my colleagues at Community Care Alliance to acknowledge my retirement.)

Acknowledgments

This book is a complete surprise to this grateful writer. I never expected that I would write something even close to a book—and yet here it is. There are many people to whom I am so grateful.

First, I acknowledge my hairdresser, Deb Fealhaber, who asked the right question at the right time. Life is so much like that. When I sat down in Debbie's chair for my haircut she asked, "So what are you up to now that you are retired?" She was the first person with whom I shared my first story. With her encouragement I wrote other stories and shared them with more people. Thanks so much for helping me to get started with this project Deb! My colleagues can attest that whenever someone at work noticed that I got a haircut my usual response was, "It's so weird that when I went for my therapy appointment last night and I came home with a haircut!" Deb has been a consistent confidant for over thirty years and a dear friend.

Secondly, I am so grateful to my brother Ron, my second confidant. Quite unexpectedly, he also became someone with whom I shared early stories. Ron also worked in the field of mental health in residential care for a number of years. His wisdom, kindness, and input were so very helpful and instrumental in growing this project. Thanks Ron!!

God is so good and loves sending surprises to us at just the opportune moment. Who would have thought that my dear altar guild buddy, Phyllis Dobbins, would have been a book editor for decades at a publishing company?? When she heard that I was writing stories, she volunteered her time and expertise to review my stories, providing her expertise and encouragement throughout the project. What a great blessing. Phyllis also has firsthand experience regarding mental illness. Her personal experiences and insights were exactly what was needed to grow the stories and make them more relatable. I am forever grateful to you Phyllis.

Thanks to the Memoir Writing Group at Lincoln Senior Center. I am so grateful to this wonderful group of writers who meet twice a month to share stories. They were such a help to improve writing skills and the stories we are putting out there. I am especially grateful to Lynn Price, the group leader and organizer. She puts so much into the group and especially into helping us to improve our skills so that the stories we write can be so much better. Thanks to all of you.

Thank you to Dr. Jim and Christine Schwarz who also took time out of their busy lives to read through the stories and send much needed input that helped to improve the stories. Your honest and sensitive input provided some perspective that improved my understanding of how to think about my work and work lessons.

Most important is my eternal gratitude to my sister Simone and our dear friend Ilona O'Connor. For hours and hours, they sat with me as we went through the stories word by word. They patiently, honestly, and lovingly provided much needed input and suggestions to help improve the stories. Both of these incredible women have had years of experience themselves working with the most vulnerable of us in this world. Because of their compassion and commitment to our most vulnerable neighbors, the stories were able to become more personal and also, more relatable to those who will read them. Thank you so very much for your contributions. I love you both so much!!

Luckily, I went to this local author event at Cumberland Public Library and met Steven Porter from Stillwater River Publications. Steve is the first publisher I have ever met. What most impressed me about him and his business is his total and unwavering commitment to supporting local authors. Thank you so much for walking me through this process inch by inch. You are the best and I cannot thank you enough for making this project a reality.

There are many others who offered encouragement and input into this project and I am grateful to all for your suggestions and support.

Finally, I am more grateful than words can convey to the many clients and colleagues who became a part of my life story and changed me in ways unimaginable over the many, many years I spent working in community mental health. What an incredible journey I have had the privilege to be a part of.

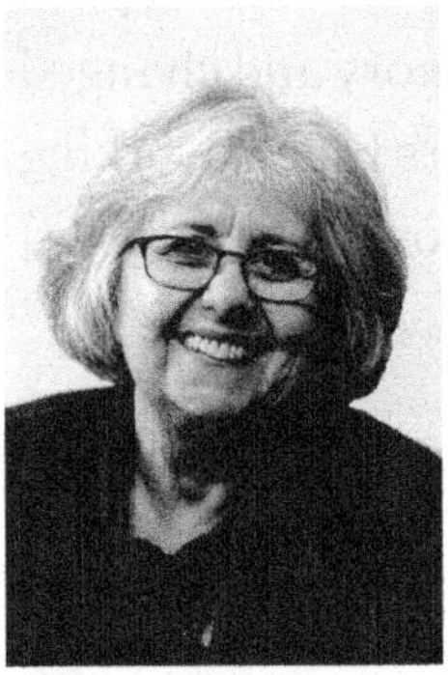

Celeste Charpentier Greene is happily retired, living in Rhode Island and enjoying spending time with friends and family, learning how to play pickleball, and being of service to her church community.

After thirty-eight years working in community mental health, stories about clients and lessons learned presented themselves and needed to be written and shared. This is her first venture into the field of authorship and publishing.

Made in the USA
Monee, IL
13 September 2026

62976615R00095